Rediscover Your
Native Fitness

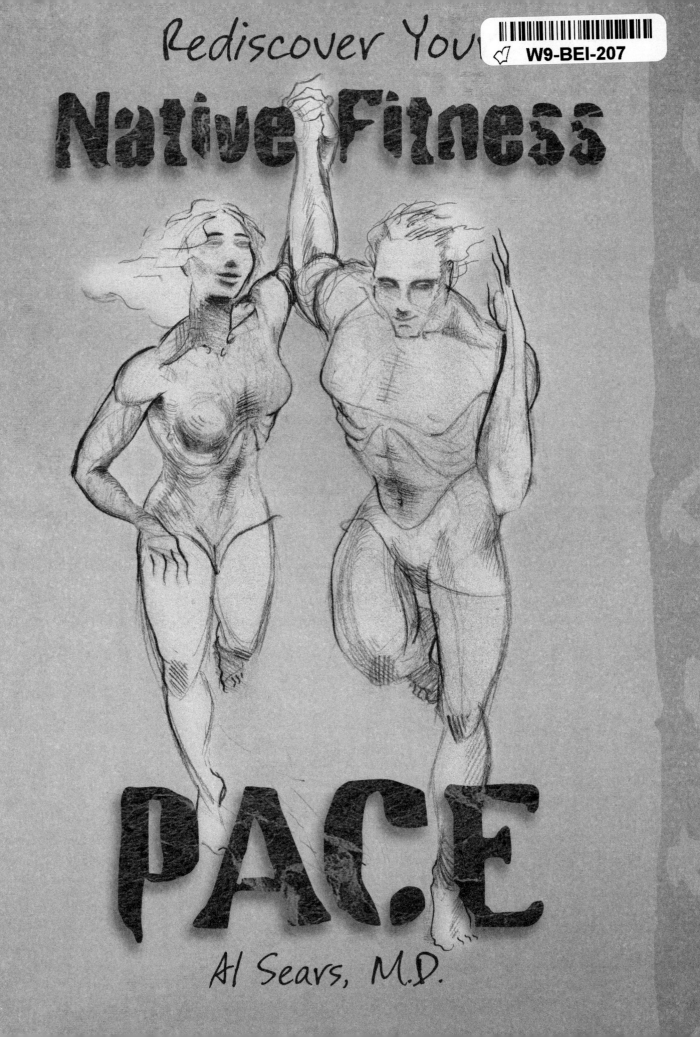

P.A.C.E

Al Sears, M.D.

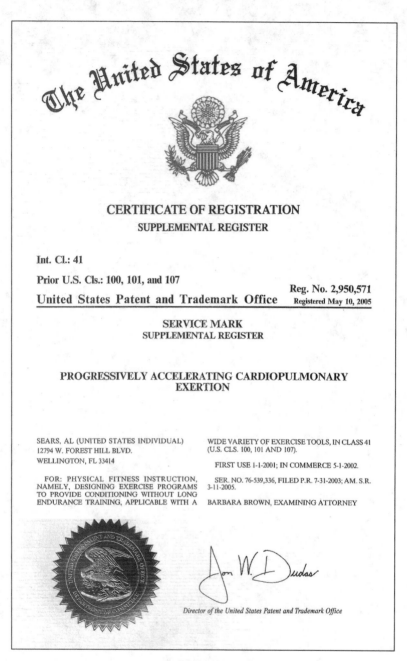

The United States of America

CERTIFICATE OF REGISTRATION
SUPPLEMENTAL REGISTER

Int. Cl.: 41

Prior U.S. Cls.: 100, 101, and 107

United States Patent and Trademark Office

Reg. No. 2,950,571
Registered May 10, 2005

SERVICE MARK
SUPPLEMENTAL REGISTER

PROGRESSIVELY ACCELERATING CARDIOPULMONARY EXERTION

SEARS, AL (UNITED STATES INDIVIDUAL)
12794 W. FOREST HILL BLVD.
WELLINGTON, FL 33414

    FOR: PHYSICAL FITNESS INSTRUCTION, NAMELY, DESIGNING EXERCISE PROGRAMS TO PROVIDE CONDITIONING WITHOUT LONG ENDURANCE TRAINING, APPLICABLE WITH A

WIDE VARIETY OF EXERCISE TOOLS, IN CLASS 41 (U.S. CLS. 100, 101 AND 107).

    FIRST USE 1-1-2001; IN COMMERCE 5-1-2002.

    SER. NO. 76-539,336, FILED P.R. 7-31-2003; AM. S.R. 3-11-2005.

BARBARA BROWN, EXAMINING ATTORNEY

Director of the United States Patent and Trademark Office

Published by:
Al Sears, MD • 12794 Forest Hill Blvd., Suite 16 • Wellington, FL 33414
www.AlSearsMD.com

This book is dedicated to my father, A.C. Sears.
He taught me, at a very young age, his system of fair play
and the value of exercise.

A very special thanks to the many patients and friends who donated their time (and their bodies) to help me develop PACE®.

CONTENTS

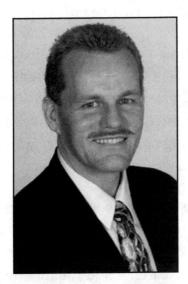

Al Sears, MD continues to see patients at his integrative clinic and research center in Florida where he has developed novel exercise and nutritional systems transforming the lives of over 20,000 patients.

He has written over 500 articles and 6 books in the fields of alternative medicine, anti-aging and nutritional supplementation. He enjoys a worldwide readership of millions spread over 123 countries, has appeared on over 50 national radio programs, ABC News, CNN and ESPN.

His third book, *The Doctor's Heart Cure*, exposed the real causes of the modern epidemic of heart disease with practical how-to advice for building real heart strength and resistance to disease without drugs. It is available in 9 languages and remains a best-seller 3 years after its publication.

In 2005, Dr. Sears' *12 Secrets to Virility* shed light on the huge environmental and nutritional problems with virility in our modern world, gave men a step-by step guide for maintaining health, strength and masculinity as they age, and became a bestseller during its first month of release.

He publishes a monthly newsletter – *Health Confidential* – addressing the issues of aging, nutrition and sexual health for men and women, a weekly e-letter called *Doctor's House Call* and is the health columnist to a circulation of hundreds of thousands in the popular self-help letter *Early to Rise*.

Dr. Sears is board certified as a clinical nutrition specialist and was appointed to the international panel of experts at **Health Sciences Institute**, (HSI) a worldwide information service for alternative nutritional therapies.

A master gardener and herbalist, Dr. Sears maintains an herbal apothecary of over 250 organic herbs used for research, education and treatments. Dr. Sears is the founder and director of The Wellness Research Foundation, conducting original research evaluating natural alternatives to pharmaceutical therapies.

Dr. Sears is a member of the American Academy of Anti-Aging Medicine and is Board Certified in Anti-Aging Medicine. As a pioneer in this new field of medicine, he is an avid researcher and sought after lecturer to thousands of doctors and health enthusiasts.

He is a member of the American College of Sports Medicine and the National Youth Sports Coaches Association. As well as being a sports and fitness coach and a lifelong advocate of exercise programs, Dr. Sears is an ACE certified fitness trainer.

Introduction

We in the modern West are out of condition but in a different way than most people think. To complicate matters, without an understanding of the cause of the problem, pundits have advocated the wrong solutions. We can divide the most popular modern exercise advice into three categories:

    1) "Cardio"
    2) Weight training and
    3) Aerobics.

All three are simply wrong and ineffective. Practice these misconceived notions long enough and they will further rob you of the native fitness you were built to enjoy.

"Cardio" has become so popular we have accepted the term as a synonym for exercise for your heart. This unfortunate misnomer is worse than a waste of your time. It only takes you further from your natural challenges and aggravates the problem. It's not natural to repeat the same movement continuously 10,000 times over without variation or rest. It will not build heart health and does not correct for what we are lacking.

Weight training is equally unnatural, ineffective and misnamed. Far from "training" anything, practicing these isolated tensing movements "untrains" your muscles. Instead of producing real strength that you can use in real situations, it produces bloated muscle fibers that become dysfunctional, injury prone and uncoupled from neuronal coordination.

Similarly, the explosion of "aerobics" classes has been associated with continued worsening of our nation's health. Its flawed and incomplete science falls to pieces under analysis. It's also poorly named because, as "cardio" won't strengthen your heart, "aerobics" won't strengthen your breath or your lungs. In fact, repeatedly exercising by "staying within your aerobic limits" will only shrink your lungs, robbing you of critical lung capacity and creating a series of other health problems.

Yet you need to do something. You are in the middle of the biggest chronic disease epidemic the world has ever known and this modern deconditioning forms its foundation. Two out of three Americans are now overweight. Diabetes is 9 times more likely than it was just 30 years ago. Heart disease kills over 1,000,000 each year in the US alone and the World Health Organization has recently announced that for the first time in history, these "chronic diseases" surpassed all other causes of death worldwide.

These new threats may attack with sudden deadly ferocity. Stroke victims rarely see it coming and half of heart attack deaths have the first symptom with the beginning of the attack that kills. Or, they may nip at your heels until their cumulative effect brings you down or you find yourself too fat, weak and tired to do anything about it. This slow degeneration has become the "status quo" of maturing in the modern world. We won the battle with the human predators of our past. Now we must face and overcome this new threat of chronic disease.

Since these diseases have changed from rare curiosities to pandemics in just a few generations, we cannot blame it on our genes. Our genes haven't changed. Since we can find powerful differences in the prevalence of these modern maladies from country to country regardless of genetic heritage, it must be coming from our environment. Most notable is the complete absence of these maladies in "primitive" native cultures.

Ironically, the key to beating our new threats may lie with recreating aspects of our primitive past. We are still perfectly adapted for a life and death struggle between predator and prey. Yet we have succeeded in completely removing ourselves from that kind of a world. As is so often the case, solving a problem presents us with a new one. No longer faced with the same physical and metabolic challenges, our own natural adaptive responses to our surroundings have got us into big trouble.

The good news is that reversing this problem is easier than you might think. You don't need to force yourself through grueling monotonous "cardio", aerobics or weight training. When you replace these strategies with activities that mimic your challenges in a natural environment, the results come much faster and easier. On top of that, it takes much less of your time; it's invigorating and it's fun to do.

This book will show you how to replace these unnatural, flawed and ineffective exercise theories with what really works. You'll:

- Build both strength and capacity in your heart and lungs.
- Avoid heart attacks and cardiovascular disease.
- Develop a powerful and disease-resistant immune system.
- Dramatically increase your energy levels.
- Burn fat like never before.

Your body will be naturally strong and resilient. You'll feel energized, motivated and ready to take on any challenge. Your muscles will be their intended size –no bigger or smaller. Your breath will be deep and focused.

These benefits are naturally YOURS. They've been lying dormant all these years – waiting for you to bring them forward.

Join me now as I introduce you to PACE® – your natural plan for health, fitness and longevity.

To Your Good Health,

Al Sears, MD

CHAPTER 1

Bust Free of the "Cardio" Myth

Look at any rack of fitness magazines and you'll see glossy covers loaded with headlines telling you to do "cardio." Go to any gym and your trainer will devote some of your time to "cardio." You probably don't like it, yet you feel compelled to comply. After all, who doesn't want a healthy heart?

Common parlance has even accepted the term "cardio" (short for cardiovascular endurance training) as synonymous with exercise for your heart. But shouldn't "heart exercise" make your heart stronger?

When you study the heart's changes from cardiovascular endurance training, you find it getting weaker in some critical capacities. These weaknesses simulate the destructive effects caused by stress and aging.

"Cardio" creates a continuous durational challenge on your heart. Usually without rest. This mimics prolonged stress in a native environment. In effect, your heart feels like it's under constant threat and attack.

Your heart adapts and responds with what are intended to be short-term survival strategies. But if you routinely perpetuate that signal of stress and attack – instead of building strength – it becomes destructive.

During twenty years of working with extremely fit athletes, patients with diseased or injured hearts and average people in between, one thing is apparent: Doing what we have come to accept as <u>"cardio" exercise is a waste of your time and effort</u>.

It doesn't build what your heart really needs. It doesn't increase your heart's ability to respond to real demands. In fact, for all your effort, you only *reduce* your ability to handle suddenly demanding events that may come your way – the last thing you want.

Yet for decades now, you've heard this advice from nearly every expert and public agency with anything to say about health. The American Medical Association, The American Heart Association, The Institutes of Medicine, even the new food pyramid from the USDA all focus on durational exercise. For instance, the Institutes of Medicine recently issued a new recommendation urging that all Americans increase the <u>duration</u> of their exercise to at least one hour every day.

You are constantly made to feel that if you could just overcome your laziness and make yourself do enough of this boring drudgery, it would solve your health problems and protect your heart. If this were true, why do very "conditioned" endurance runners drop dead of heart attacks at the height of their running careers?

All that "Heart Conditioning"... Only to Drop Dead

This unfortunate "side effect" appears linked to the birth of long-distance running. We get the name "marathon" from the ancient Greek long-distance messenger, Phidippides. He famously ran 26.2 miles from Marathon to Athens to tell of the victory of the Greeks over the invading Persians. On his arrival, he announced "Nike!" (Victory) then collapsed and died.[1]

My first personal experience with this occurred 25 years ago. I was providing emergency care for a long distance race in Tampa, Florida. I saw a thin young man collapse to the ground just yards from our emergency aid station. His heart continued to violently race, as we put an oxygen mask over his blue lips. Another runner in his 20's made it to our station but had to kneel down to wait for emergency assistance. He was weak, dizzy and frightened – with a dangerously irregular heartbeat.

In the early 1980s, Jack Kelly famously suffered this same "paradoxical" fate. Jack was the brother of actress Grace Kelly. He was also an Olympic oarsman and a very accomplished distance runner. He went out for his usual morning run and, shortly after, dropped dead of sudden heart failure. At the time, he was the president of the US Olympic Committee.

Later I came to call this pattern the "Jim Fixx Phenomenon," after the popular fitness guru of the 70's. Fixx claimed that the secret to heart health and long life was endurance running – up until he died of a heart attack – while running.

I later came to realize that this happens because adding repeated "cardio" to our busy days and pushing for greater endurance produces the *opposite* physical result of what we really need in the modern world.

Look at "Cardio" from Your Heart's Perspective

Routinely forcing your body to perform the same continuous cardiovascular challenge, by repeating the same movement, at the same rate, thousands of times over, without variation, and without rest, is unnatural. This type of demand could have occurred rarely, but not in the daily environment of native societies in balance with their surroundings.

Yet nature has designed your body to adapt to whatever environment you encounter. If you ask it to perform this activity repeatedly and routinely, it will gradually change the systems involved to meet the challenge more effectively. But what adaptive changes does this activity cause?

To help answer that question, think of your body as an engine with the nifty additional feature of being able to gradually redesign itself. If you require this engine to repeatedly go non-stop for long distances against low resistance, at a relatively slow speed, its primary adaptation will be to become more efficient at light, long, continuous, low output.

Continuous duration taxing your endurance produces some unique challenges your body must overcome. It must not run out of fuel, overheat, or be overwhelmed with metabolic wastes. One of the ways that your body adapts is by gradually rebuilding your heart, lungs, blood vessels and muscles as small as possible and still have the minimum "horsepower" required.

You wouldn't build a Formula-1 car to drive in a school zone. You'd waste fuel with a Ferrari sized engine going 20 miles per hour. And you'd waste raw material to build and maintain a monster truck if you don't carry heavy loads.

Forced, continuous, endurance exercise induces your heart and lungs to "downsize" because smaller allows you to go further... more efficiently... with less rest... and less fuel.

The Danger of "Downsizing" Your Heart's Capacity

So what's wrong with increasing durational capacity through downsizing? Instead of building heart strength, it robs it of vital *reserve capacity*. Your heart's reserve capacity is that portion of its maximal output that you don't use during usual activity. To reuse the car analogy, your reserve capacity is the "pedal" that you have left on your accelerator before you hit the floorboard when you're cruising at your typical speed.

So if you downsize your heart and lungs you have traded reserve capacity for efficiency at continuous duration. This then forces them to operate dangerously close to their maximal output when circumstances challenge them. For your heart, this is a problem you don't need.

Heart attacks don't occur because of a lack of endurance. They occur when there is a sudden increase in cardiac demand that exceeds your heart's capacity. Giving up your heart's reserve capacity to adapt to unnatural bouts of continuous prolonged duration only increases your risk of sudden cardiac death.

A ground-breaking study of long-distance runners showed that after a workout, the blood levels and oxidation of LDL (bad) cholesterol and triglycerides increased. They also found that prolonged running disrupted the balance of blood thinners and thickeners, elevating inflammatory factors and clotting levels – both signs of heart distress.[2]

And it's bad for your bones too. A study published in the Journal of Clinical Endocrinology & Metabolism found that long-distance runners had reduced bone mass. This is true for both men and women – although women had an increased risk for osteoporosis as well.[3]

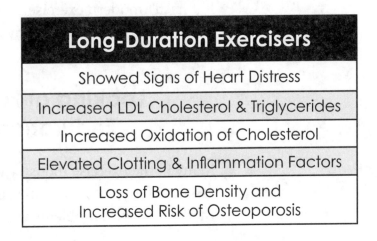

Long-Duration Exercisers
Showed Signs of Heart Distress
Increased LDL Cholesterol & Triglycerides
Increased Oxidation of Cholesterol
Elevated Clotting & Inflammation Factors
Loss of Bone Density and Increased Risk of Osteoporosis

These changes do not reflect a heart that's becoming stronger after exercise. And many of the subjects in this study stopped the exercise complaining of boredom.

Exercising for long periods makes your heart adept at handling a 60-minute jog, but it accomplishes this by trading in its ability to rapidly provide you with big bursts when circumstances might demand.

The real key to prevent heart disease and protect and strengthen your heart is to induce the opposite adaptive response produced by continuous cardio and increase your heart's reserve capacity. Bigger, faster cardiac output more immediately available is what you really need.

Recent clinical studies show us the benefit of avoiding long-duration routines and exercising in shorter bursts. Researchers from the University of Missouri found that short bouts of exercise were more effective for lowering fat and triglyceride levels in the blood.[4] (High triglycerides dramatically increase your risk of heart disease.)

Another study revealed that the **duration** of exercise routines predicts the risk of heart disease in men. They found that several shorter sessions of physical activity were more effective for lowering the risk of coronary heart disease.[5]

But hasn't modern exercise science proven that "cardio" is the best way to get rid of body fat? Actually, it's also a poor tool for getting lean.

Looking at Fat as Fuel for Endurance Exercise

Many in the exercise industry will tell you that "cardio" is essential for you to burn off your body fat and get lean. Yet there are several problems with this exercise theory.

For starters, consider the experience of body builders. Many of the very leanest people in this sport (some of the leanest people on the planet in fact) insist that part of their secret to getting and staying lean is: "Never do cardio."

My patient, John D, a world-class bodybuilder, is a staunch advocate of "no cardio." He, like many others in his field, told me that avoiding cardio is the only way to keep your muscle while getting extremely lean.

Science backs him up on this too. A new study shows that the muscles of marathon runners actually shrink. When the muscle biopsies of marathon runners were analyzed, researchers found their muscle fiber size had decreased and atrophied.[6]

This is not to advocate body building, but when someone 280 pounds with the incredibly low body fat of 4% reports that he got that lean while avoiding "cardio" and performing "reps" of exertion lasting 2 seconds in "sets" lasting less than 1 minute, it raises an interesting question about duration of exercise exertion and body fat.

And what about the comparison of native hunters to native farmers? Hunters spend less energy in shorter duration bouts but have nearly universally lower body fat than farmers who spend hours of durational exertion in the fields all day. Many factors could account for this observation. But again, the association of shorter exertion with lower body fat raises interests to investigate.

Don't you have to exercise for at least 15 or 20 minutes before you really kick into fat burning mode? Well, sort of... but there's more to it than that.

Your body can select from several fuel sources. It can burn fat, it can burn carbohydrates like glycogen or it can get energy from breaking down protein. When you exercise for different durations or at different levels of intensity it alters the relative proportion of energy you derive from these 3 sources.

For the first couple of minutes, your body uses something called ATP – the most readily available source of energy.

But your supplies of ATP are limited. After 2 to 3 minutes, your body switches to carbs stored in muscle tissue. This lasts for 15 to 20 minutes before you switch to fat.

As you'll see, this means that your PACE® routines are very short – never lasting for more than 15 to 20 minutes. But your body makes fuel choices based on your activity level as well…

Look at the following table.

Body Fuel with Varying Activity			
Activity Level	**Protein**	**Carbs**	**Fat**
Resting	1 - 5%	35%	60%
Low Intensity	5 - 8%	70%	15%
Moderate Intensity	2 - 5%	40%	55%
High Intensity	2%	95%	3%

Adapted from: McArdle W.D. 1999. Sports & Exercise Nutrition. NY: Lippincott Williams & Wilkins

From reviewing the chart, you see that at low intensity activity your body derives most of its energy from carbohydrate and only 15% from fat. When you look at the lifestyle of our ancient ancestors, this makes sense. Low intensity activity – like walking long distances – was natural for hunter-gatherers. Still today, long walks are health-enhancing activities and as Henry David Thoreau said, "Walking is exercise for the soul."

But when you step up your activity level to moderate, you increase the percentage of the energy burned from fat to 55% of the total. Now notice that if you increase your activity to high intensity you dramatically reduce your dependency on fat and derive nearly all your energy from carbs.

This relationship has lead many to advise that you should exercise at moderate intensity because that's how you burn the most fat. Although this seems logical, it turns out to be completely the wrong advice for getting lean.

To help explain, remember the analogy of your body as an engine but with that added feature of being capable of changing itself to better meet recurrent demands. What adaptive response do you induce by burning fat as your principle fuel? Your body will build more fat to better prepare itself for this activity.

All That Time and Effort... to Build More Fat

Burning fat while exercising signals to your body that it needed the fat. <u>This trains your body to make more fat for the next time you exercise</u>. Your body then replenishes your fat each time you eat and becomes efficient at building and preserving fat necessary for long mid-level cardiovascular sessions in preparation for the next endurance workout. In doing so, it sacrifices muscle and other high-energy burning tissues and preserves fat.

So don't bother trying to use this strategy to lose body fat. Your body will fight you in the effort and you can only do it by sacrificing lean tissue like muscle and internal organs.

And if the sole purpose of the activity was to maximize the proportion of energy derived from fat, why not just rest? Notice from the table that the body burns an even higher percentage of energy as fat (60%) <u>while resting</u>. The "cardio" proponents seem to overlook this fact.

So durational exercise stimulates your body to build fat. Then, if you stop your "cardio," you'll put on fat very rapidly. And many find they have to stop because this unnatural activity has caused degeneration of their joints.

And another point: If you persist through middle age and beyond, it accelerates some very negative effects of aging. It lowers testosterone and growth hormone, boosts destructive cortisol levels and robs you of muscle, bone and internal organ mass and strength.

<u>While short duration exercise actually increases levels of growth hormone</u>. Researchers from Loughborough University in Leicestershire, England tested growth hormone levels in sprinters and endurance athletes. On average, the sprinters had 3 times as much growth hormone as the endurance runners.[7]

But the biggest point is this: The most important changes from exercise occur after, not during, the exercise period. The way you exercise affects your metabolism for several days. The important changes begin <u>after you stop exercising</u>. This is good news. It means that all you have to do during your exercise is to stimulate the adaptive response you need. Then, your body will continue making the important changes afterwards – while you rest.

Signal Your Body to Build What It Lacks

Short bursts of exercise tell your body that storing energy as fat is inefficient, since you never exercise long enough to utilize the fat during each session. Carbohydrates, which are stored in muscle rather than fat, burn energy at high rates. Exercising for short periods will use these carbs and burn much more fat after exercising while you replenish the carbs. Short interval exercise maximizes fat "after burn."

Researchers at Laval University in Quebec divided participants into two groups: long-duration and repeated short-duration exercisers.[8] They had the long-duration group cycle 45 minutes without interruption. The short-term interval group cycled in numerous short bursts of 15 – 90 seconds, while resting in between.

The long duration group burned twice as many calories, so you would assume they would burn more fat. However, when the researchers recorded their body composition measurements, the interval group showed that they lost the most fat.

In fact, the interval group **lost 9 times more fat** than the endurance group for every calorie burned. Doesn't this defy the laws of physics? No, it just illustrates that exercise continues to affect your metabolism after you stop. The short bursts stimulated a greater after burn.

In addition, short duration bursts produce many other desirable results for your metabolic health:

- Improves maximal cardiac outputs.

- Promotes the development of quicker cardiac adjustments to changes in demand.

- Helps you lose body fat with as little as 10 minutes per day.

- Achieves "higher peak stroke volumes during overload." (Your peak stroke volume is the maximal amount of blood your heart can pump per beat when maximally challenged.)

- Improves cholesterol levels, (subjects in a study of exercise bursts showed a decrease in total cholesterol and an increase in "good" cholesterol).[9]

- Provides an anti-aging benefit by raising testosterone levels, which fights against memory loss, accumulation of fat, low libido, sexual dysfunction, and loss of strength and bone.[10]

- Helps you lose weight by burning much more fat after you stop exercising.

And, you'll be able to get these benefits with much less of your time – no need to spend hours at the gym.

So the recent "cardio craze" was a mistake because it produces an unnatural challenge and failed to take into account your body's adaptive responses like shrinking internal organs, shrinking and weakening muscles, decreased cardiac reserve capacity and an increased dependency on body fat for energy. But don't you still need an "aerobics" workout for your lungs?

As you'll see in the next chapter, if you want to be lean, energetic, disease-free and injury resistant, while building powerful lungs, forget about modern aerobics and rediscover native "supra-aerobics."

CHAPTER 2

Beyond "Aerobics" - Rediscover Your Native Fat Burner

You've seen that continuous durational exercise like what we refer to as "cardio" mimics stress causing you to grow weaker in some vitally important capacities. Now let's look at the related exercise characteristic of intensity of your effort, how this applies to the phenomenon of aerobics, and the adaptive response generated.

Let's get back to our car analogy. A small engine might be fine for long road trips. But if you need extra power fast, you're in trouble. As you've read, your heart and lungs are analogous. By doing durational cardio, you're actually making your heart and lungs smaller so they can withstand long-duration workouts. But as a result, you lose your reserve capacity – the ability to get extra power fast.

Think of this concept of extra power as the "turbo" in your car. You probably won't need that turbo power in normal traffic. But if someone is chasing you, and you need to make a quick getaway, that turbo will save your life by giving you that extra power right at the moment you need it.

So when it comes to exercise, it's a good idea to build and strengthen your "turbo power." You make sure your heart and lungs have the ability to generate lots of power very quickly – just in case. Access to extra power is what our ancient ancestors built and maintained naturally in their native environment. But it's lacking in our modern world. PACE® is a safe, easy and reliable way to rebuild your **high-energy output system**.

So if this **high-energy output system** is key, let's look at what happens when we focus on training our oxygen delivering power with "aerobics".

Back in the late 1960s, Dr. Kenneth Cooper published *Aerobics* as the "perfect" way to "train" your heart and boost your aerobic conditioning. He thought that medium intensity aerobic exercise practiced three or four times a week was all you needed for health and longevity.

Yet this theory was never really proven and recently the pieces are crumbling under the weight of mounting evidence to the contrary. For instance, a recent study by Harvard researchers shows that those who do short-duration, high-intensity workouts, reduce their risk of heart disease by ***100 percent more*** than those who practice aerobic exercise.[1]

A study published in the *Archives of Internal Medicine* showed that men and women who exercised at a higher intensity had lower blood pressure, lower triglycerides (blood fat), higher HDL (good cholesterol) and less body fat.[2]

What's more, medium intensity does not train your high-energy output system – or to refer back to your car – your turbo system. To do that, you need to kick it up a notch and do a higher intensity routine. Not coincidentally, you are only capable of doing this <u>for a shorter length of time</u> than advocated by aerobics theory.

Forget Aerobics – Discover Your *REAL* Fat-Burning Zone

A few years ago, a patient of mine – BP – came to me very deconditioned and getting old before his time. He said his cardiologist told him to never exceed his "aerobic threshold" when he exercised. But if you never exceed your current aerobic capacity you will never signal your body to increase your aerobic capacity and your aerobic deconditioning will surely persist and eventually worsen. Only by exceeding your aerobic capacity, will you encourage your body to increase lung strength.

To better understand what your aerobic threshold is, we need to take a closer look at metabolism...

Metabolism is simply how the cells in your body process different substances to obtain energy. In your muscles, ATP is the molecule they use for energy. You use 2 different systems in your cells to generate ATP, aerobic and anaerobic.

ATP molecules are the basic unit of cellular energy. It's the first source of energy your muscles use. But you don't have a lot of ATP on hand at any given time. After a few seconds, you have to replace the ATP burned if you want to continue activities. The more you exert yourself, the more ATP your body needs to make.

Let's say you're walking down the street. At first, your body will use available ATP to feed your muscle cells. Then to replenish ATP, your body kicks in its aerobic metabolism.

Aerobic means "with oxygen." So your aerobic metabolism combines oxygen with carbs, fats and proteins to make ATP. Because walking is not a strenuous activity, you can easily obtain enough oxygen to make all the ATP you need. Using this model, you could walk for hours and not run out of fuel and not feel too tired.

But let's say you start jogging. The faster pace requires more energy. That means your cells will use oxygen more quickly. To keep the system working, you have to breathe harder to get more oxygen into your cells. At the same time, your heart starts to beat faster in order to get the oxygen to muscle cells more quickly.

Jogging is a typical aerobic exercise because it can be sustained with oxygen metabolism (aerobic metabolism). But what happens when your body can't get enough oxygen from aerobic metabolism alone?

To answer that, let's say you start sprinting. For the first 5 or 10 seconds, you can sustain that high output with oxygen – but not for much longer. You can't produce ATP with oxygen as fast as you are using it and your muscles start to become ATP depleted. <u>That's the point at which your anaerobic energy system kicks in</u>. This is also known as crossing your **aerobic threshold**.

Anaerobic means "without oxygen." This system converts carbs – and some fats – into energy without using oxygen. This will sustain you in a sprint for a while. You can get a very high-energy output from this system but not for very long. And you'll notice that when you stop sprinting you will continue to pant heavily for oxygen.

Panting means that you've created an *oxygen debt*. This occurs when your muscles ask for more oxygen than your lungs can supply at that moment – like when you're sprinting.

Understanding when the anaerobic system kicks in is critical. When you're using your anaerobic system, you are training your <u>high-energy output system</u>.

When this happens, you are successfully building up reserve capacity in your heart, expanding your lung volume, triggering the production of growth hormone and melting away fat.

And all these years, doctors, trainers and fitness "gurus" believing in the aerobics myth have been telling us to never cross that aerobic threshold!

But let's take this a step further... And this is the big misunderstanding that I want to set straight: <u>Aerobic and anaerobic can only be used to describe metabolism</u>. Like in the above description.

Aerobic and anaerobic just doesn't apply to exercise. This is where modern exercise science has steered us in the wrong direction. It's possible for your cells to make energy without oxygen – but it's impossible for you to exercise without oxygen – even if you hold your breath.

In essence, there's no such thing as anaerobic exercise. When you're sprinting, your body will start its anaerobic metabolism, but you are still using oxygen for the exercise. In fact, when your anaerobic system kicks in, your aerobic system is still functioning. One does not replace the other.

Aerobic energy production is simply limited in how much energy it can produce per time. If you exceed that rate, you will continue to produce the maximum energy you are capable of with aerobic metabolism. But now you will add more energy from your anaerobic energy system.

So the term anaerobic exercise really makes no sense. It's more appropriate to say that you've exceeded your aerobic limit and crossed over into your **supra-aerobic zone**.

By shedding this aerobics dogma and training yourself into your **supra-aerobic zone**, you're going to restore native health benefits amazingly fast: A bulletproof heart, powerful lungs, strong muscles, youthful features, no excess fat and a long life.

Your Ancient Ancestors Used their "Supra-Aerobic Zone"

Until recent times – and until "experts" told us not to – we have always, at times, exerted ourselves with extreme intensity and purpose. All animals are either predator or prey. In the case of the human animal, we were both. We still have the genetic make-up to respond to the challenge – and we need to.

As my insightful colleague, Dr Phil Goscienski put it in his *Health Secrets of the Stone Age*:

"Most modern humans do not exercise as if their lives depended on it – but they do… If we don't push our heart and lungs toward their limits they will have little reserve, incapable of meeting the demands of stress, infection or injury."

"Thousands of generations ago (we) may have become another creatures meal… Now …(we) are just as surely killed by diseases that were almost nonexistent, even in the elderly, back in prehistory. Instead of death that came in seconds, however grisly those last seconds must have been, our dying takes years."[3]

Downsizing Your Lungs – Like Your Heart – Can Have Disastrous Consequences

In the last chapter, you learned how traditional "cardio" downsizes your heart and makes it lose vital reserve capacity. Aerobics practiced regularly will similarly shrink your lungs as well.

I first observed and documented this when I was an undergraduate in college. I always wanted to be a gymnast but I wasn't that good in tumbling routines. But I could do the strength moves better than anyone on the team.

The coach asked me how I developed shoulder, arm and back strength. When I told him that I didn't lift weights he asked me to assist in strength training the team. I had a job at the school infirmary so I borrowed the use of their equipment to measure as many parameters of strength that I could. This would be our starting point.

As part of this assessment, I ran a series of pulmonary function tests. I put those with the lowest lung volumes into running programs because everyone "knew" that long distance running would make you develop more lungpower.

A few months later, after they had finished a long-duration cardio program, I ran another series of lung capacity tests. Much to my initial shock, their lung capacity had shrunk. That's when it all began to click...

If you don't challenge your maximal capacity – like when you enter your supra-aerobic zone – you'll actually give up lung capacity. What's more, the strain accelerates your loss of lung volume and speeds up the aging process – making you even more vulnerable to infection and chronic disease.

PACE®, on the other hand, challenges your peak lung volume. When you exercise in your supra-aerobic zone – and create an oxygen debt – you send a signal to your lungs to expand. Over time, your body adapts to the challenge by increasing its lung volume and power.

Over the years, I've seen remarkable results in my own patients. PACE® has helped people across the board. From asthmatics to die-hard smokers, the effects of PACE® have reversed long-term damage and restored healthy lungpower in hundreds of cases.

For years, Dr. Izumi Tabata has been working on similar research at the National Institute of Health and Nutrition in Tokyo, Japan. His most famous study shows the powerful effects that short, high-intensity workouts can have on your lungs.

He measured the VO_2 Max (the amount of oxygen that gets transported to cells in a given amount of time), and the anaerobic capacity of two groups of cyclists. One group did medium-intensity long duration routines – like aerobics – and the other did short, high-intensity routines – like PACE®.

After six weeks, the group doing the short, high-intensity workouts improved their VO_2 Max by 14 percent and their anaerobic capacity by a remarkable 28 percent.[4]

This means that the high-intensity workouts not only improved their lung volume, but also raised the amount of oxygen their body could produce during their workouts. This performance boost enabled them to hit their supra-aerobic zone and trigger the adaptive responses that create a lean, disease-free body. And you only have to achieve this level for a minute or so to produce results.

Lactic Acid is Not Your Enemy… It's Fuel

Finally, one of the last "old theories" of aerobic training is crumbling under the weight of new evidence. At the center of the breakthrough is *lactic acid*.

You've probably heard of it, especially if you've ever had a coach or a trainer. Conventional wisdom said you had to avoid lactic acid because its build up in your muscles caused pain, fatigue and the soreness you feel after "over doing it."

We were told to exercise aerobically and not cross the dreaded **lactic threshold**. Lactic acid starts to build in the muscles when your anaerobic system kicks in. The idea that you had to avoid lactic acid helped to spur the aerobics craze that reached its peak in the 1980's.

But this theory never jived with the real world experience of the benefits of exceeding your aerobic threshold (which would build lots of the dreaded lactic acid). It turns out lactic acid is **not your enemy**. To the contrary, it's fuel for your muscles.

Dr. George Brooks from the University of California at Berkeley recently found that lactic acid is taken up and burned for energy by your mitochondria – the energy factories in your muscle cells.[5] What's more, it cannot create the after workout soreness because it is rapidly removed as you burn it for fuel. In other words, it's long gone before you get sore.

A high output, supra-aerobic workout is exactly what your body needs to increase your lungpower, build reserve capacity in your heart and melt away your fat stores.

Remember... aerobic exercise is low to medium output held for an extended period. Supra-aerobic exercise is high output, but short in duration. Why is this important? For one thing, it restores an element of your native environment.

Our ancestors lived in a world where their food fought back. Predators attacked without notice. They had to run or fight – fast and hard. These short bursts of high-output activity fine tuned our ancient ancestors and kept them fit. We still have the same physiology yet have lost that kind of challenge.

To move your workout into the anaerobic range, the key feature is this: Create an "oxygen debt" as I described earlier. Simply exercise at a pace you can't sustain for more than a short period. Ask your lungs for more oxygen than they can provide.

The difference between the oxygen you need and the oxygen you get is your oxygen debt. This will cause you to pant and continue to breathe hard even after you've stopped the exertion until you replace the oxygen you're lacking.

Here's another example: Let's say you pedal as fast as you can on a bike for 15 seconds. When you stop, you continue to pant. This is the kind of high-output challenge you can't sustain for very long. You have reached your *supra-aerobic zone*. This is very different from doing an aerobic workout for 45 minutes.

This is the basis for your PACE® program. I began using most of this program 25 years ago. More recently, I added progressivity to increase the benefits.

By making small changes in the same direction, your workouts can produce remarkable results. And you only need 12 minutes to achieve the desired effect.

In a matter of weeks, you can:

- Lose pounds of belly fat

- Build functional new muscle

- Reverse heart disease

- Build energy reserves available on demand

- Strengthen your immune system

- Reverse many of the changes of aging.

Remember the *Real* Secret Behind Fat Burning!

If you want to see the fat melt off your body, you must achieve supra-aerobic performance levels with your PACE® program.

How do you know if you are doing this?

Simple. Monitor your heart rate while you're doing PACE®. When you finish an intense interval, you should see your heart rate go up a few points immediately after you slow down. If you do this successfully, you will feel yourself start to pant.

But don't worry. Heavy breathing for a few moments is a good thing. It means that you're demanding more oxygen from your body than it can provide at that particular moment.

This is an oxygen deficit. It's the essence of supra-aerobic exercise. While panting is tiring, it's the best thing you can do and you don't have to do it for very long.

With short bursts of intense exercise, your body burns the energy stored in muscle tissue, instead of energy stored as fat. This teaches your body to store more energy in the muscles – not as fat – so it's available for quick bursts of energy.

PACE® stands for <u>P</u>rogressively <u>A</u>ccelerating <u>C</u>ardiopulmonary <u>E</u>xertion. The PACE® program starts with interval training, but takes it a step further. Let's look at how these principles are unique to PACE® and how they work together to create a healthy heart and a fat-free body.

Progressivity – Repeated Changes in the Same Direction

Exercise is much more effective when you do a little more of one component each time you do it. <u>Progressivity is repeated changes in the same direction</u>. Rather than exercising for longer periods, you increase your intensity levels. As your heart capacity increases, you should add resistance or pick up your pace gradually.

Progressivity is also the need to change your routine over time (more on this later). Doing the same routine over and over – whether cardio or weight training – will lead to failure. Your body needs a consistent set of new challenges in order to grow and achieve.

These changes – made over time – embody the concept of **progressivity**.

Acceleration – Adapting Faster to Demands

As you train your body to respond faster each time you exercise, your physical condition improves. Then, as your body responds more quickly – by increasing your pace, or the resistance, in each progressive workout session – it adapts to the demands. This is the principle of **acceleration.**

It is the best way to gear up for unexpected increases in cardiac demands.

When you first begin exercising, it will take several minutes to get your heart rate and breathing up. This is your low cardiopulmonary capacity, or de-conditioned phase. But as you begin moving at a faster pace, you'll condition yourself to meet the challenge.

By starting at a comfortable exercise level, you'll enhance your response capacity by increasing your pace sooner in each workout as you progress. The quickness of the demand each time accelerates the development of your adaptive capacity.

This experience tells your body that it needs to increase your lung volume in order to deal with the increased demand for oxygen. It also builds the critical reserve capacity your heart needs to function at its strongest.

Lung volume and reserve capacity are two key principles of anti-aging. By creating an oxygen deficit after each interval, you are building the body of a warrior. A body that <u>builds muscle and burns fat</u>.

In addition, the oxygen deficit tells your body to burn the glycogen stored in your muscle as fuel. This is essential for fat burning. As you are beginning to see, fat burning happens after you finish your workout. Why?

If you burn glycogen (a form of carbohydrate) while you exercise, your body will burn fat after the workout in order to restore its fuel levels in your muscle tissue. If you do this repeatedly, your body becomes used to burning fat after each workout.

As you'll see, PACE® puts your body into fat burning mode – automatically!

Dream Body Revealed:
One Man's Amazing Journey

Just ask MF. He gave me permission to share his statistics and progress with you, as further proof of the PACE® program's positive results.

When Mike first visited me, he had 50% body fat and took 11 drugs for his physical problems. In just **12 weeks**, he lowered his body fat to 30%... and in **18 months**, Mike achieved a body fat score of 10%.

As you can see from the chart below, Mike also lost 66 pounds from February 2002 to April 2003. What's more, he threw away the prescriptions for the 11 drugs he was taking.

Date	02-08-02	04-22-02	02-05-03	04-29-03
Weight	283	263	226	217
Skin Fold				
Chest	48	30	10	6
Abdomen	60	42	12	8
Thigh	50	30	20	14
TOTAL	158	102	42	28
% Body Fat	42%	31%	14.4%	10%
Pounds of Fat	119	82	33	22
Lean Body Mass	164	181	193	195

Mike Before and After PACE®

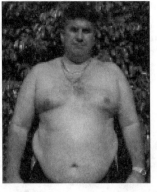
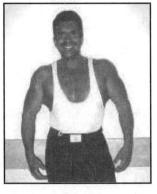

CHAPTER 3

Jumpstart Your PACE® Now!

So now, you know the basics of my very different approach to fitness. You're excited about PACE®, but don't know where to start. I suggest you start with the simple and easy 10-minute workout below.

Your goal is to slightly tax you heart, lungs, blood vessels and muscles with cardiopulmonary exertion. In other words, you want to give your ability to deliver oxygen and fuel to your muscles a good workout. You can use various exercises or machines to give your heart and lungs a challenge, depending on your fitness level.

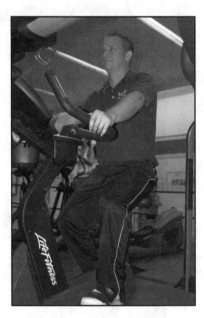

PACE® is very flexible. Whether you like the gym or prefer the outdoors, PACE® can adapt to any environment. Indoors, you can do your PACE® workout on a stationary bike, recumbent bike, elliptical, stair-stepper or treadmill. Outdoors, you can run, swim or ride your bike.

This easy, 10-minute workout is very straightforward. For now, you're NOT going to apply all of the principles you learned in the last chapter. To get started, you're just going to begin with simple sets of exertion and recovery.

Use caution and always check with your doctor before starting this or any exercise program. Especially if any of the following factors on the next page apply to you:

> **Doctor's Tip**:
>
> If you're over 65, obese or out of shape, you can still do PACE. Even if you feel like you can't run, you can still do what I call "walking PACE®".
>
> During your first exertion period walk at a brisk pace, something that's easy but gives you a challenge. When you hit your recovery, rest and feel your heart rate slow down. Then repeat. It's that easy!

Risk Factors
Over 50 Years Old
No Medical Checkup Within Two Years
25+ Pounds Overweight
High Blood Pressure
Heart Attack, Rapid Heart Palpitations, Chest Pain After Exercise
Taking Heart Medication
Angina, Fibrillation, Tachycardia, Abnormal EKG, Heart Murmur, Rheumatic Heart Disease
Blood Relative Died From Heart Attack Before Age 60
Asthma, Emphysema, or another Lung Condition

** **Note:** When beginning an exercise program, it's important to start out light and increase your effort over time.

Start Here:
The 10-Minute Program Chart

<u>This program is simply alternating between periods of exertion and recovery</u>.

Set 1		Set 2		Set 3		Set 4		Set 5	
Exertion	Recovery	Exert.	Rec.	Exert.	Rec.	Exert.	Rec.	Exert.	Rec.
1 min	1 min	1 min	1 min	1 min	1 min	1 min	1 min	1 min	1 min

I refer to each period of exertion followed by recovery as one set. I will be referring to these throughout the book. Now let's use this simple 10-minute program to get a better idea of how it works.

Look at the program chart above. Your first minute is a period of exertion. For the first sixty seconds, you're going to exercise at a pace that gives your heart and lungs a challenge.

If you're new to exercise, or feel out-of-shape, take it easy for the first two weeks. The speed and intensity of your exertion should be fast enough for you to break a sweat, but not so intense that you have any trouble finishing the 10-minute program.

After your first exertion period, begin your first recovery period. During your recovery period, slow down to an easy pace – as if you're walking. <u>You don't need to stop moving during your recovery.</u> Simply slow down and go at a slow, easy speed. Focus on normalizing your breathing and tell your mind and body to relax. This gives your body a chance to rest and recover. In this way, you train your ability to recover from exertion and stress.

Now that you have a feel for it in your first set, simply repeat the process for your second set. Start your next exertion period and follow it with a recovery period. You'll soon get into the groove of exercising in short bursts followed by periods of recovery.

Getting your feet wet with simple exertion and recovery training will help you get started right away. What's more, it will prepare you for the PACE® program, which builds on this kind of interval training by adding other dimensions like progressivity, incremental intensity, decreasing duration and acceleration.

At this stage, you're taking on new ideas and new challenges and giving your body a chance to adapt. And this **_adaptive response_** is critical for change and advancement.

Modern science tends to view your body as a lifeless machine. If something breaks down, simply replace the part and move on. But your body is a living organism with its own sense of timing, intelligence and connection to its

Doctor's Tip:

Keep a journal of your PACE® workouts. Writing down your goals, plans and the details of your workouts will keep you focused and motivated. What's more, it will enable you to see and measure your progress. Take a moment each time and jot down your numbers. If you don't, you won't know how much fat you've lost!

environment. Your body makes decisions based on what you subject it too. It can think, react and make changes.

The PACE® program works with your body. By giving it the right set of challenges, it enables your body to make adaptive responses that result in weight loss, fat burning and a build up of reserve capacity in your heart and lungs.

This gives you the opportunity to transform your body – no matter how overweight or out-of-shape you were when you started. By starting with this simple 10-minute workout and giving your body new challenges over time, you can burn fat like a champion – guaranteed. And you'll avoid the chronic diseases that kill millions every year.

PACE® Program Boosts Your Body's "Fountain of Youth" Hormone

PACE® training is far superior to traditional "cardio." New research has uncovered startling changes that take place in your body within hours of starting. (I've seen these same results in my own patients.)

Here are just a few of the added benefits:[1]

- **Raise Your Levels of Human Growth Hormone (HGH):** HGH is your body's "anti-aging" hormone. It's been clinically proven to build muscle, burn fat, improve bone density, raise your 'good' cholesterol and reverse the negative effects of aging. Blood levels of HGH rise dramatically during and immediately after. (Traditional aerobic exercise has no effect on HGH.)

- **Burn More Calories:** PACE® turbo-charges your metabolism. After intense bursts of exercise, your body needs to burn extra calories to repair muscles, replenish energy and bring your body back to its "normal" state. This process takes anywhere from a few hours up to a whole day – meaning you'll burn calories long after your workout is over.

- **Tap the Strength of Large Muscle Fibers:** Regular aerobic exercise uses smaller muscle fibers, as these fibers are more oxygen efficient. PACE® draws upon larger muscle fibers, which generate more power but get tired more easily. Moderate aerobic workouts tend to ignore these larger fibers, leaving them weak and shrunken. By exercising these larger muscle fibers, you get stronger muscles that can handle heavy-duty demands. (Critical for mobility and independence as you get older…)

- **More Strength, Greater Fitness in Less Time:** After a few weeks of a "cardio" routine, you stop making progress and hit a "plateau." PACE® helps you break through those dead spots and keeps you moving forward. Within just a few months of PACE®, you'll be able to pump more blood and deliver more oxygen to your muscles – raising your energy levels like never before.

- **Bigger, Stronger Heart:** The PACE® program gives your heart a boost you'll never get from traditional aerobic exercise. Because PACE® demands more oxygen, your heart adapts by increasing both its heart rate and stroke volume (the amount of blood your heart can pump in one beat). This increased pumping power makes your heart stronger – and last longer.

Additional Features Unique to Your PACE® Program

One thing you must do differently from previous standard exercise routines is to decrease the length of time for each exercise interval. As your conditioning increases, you will use shorter and shorter episodes of gradually increasing intensity.

Doctor's Tip:

Water is excellent for the body and good health. Water helps flush out toxins and other unwanted things lingering in the body.

Water also replenishes fluids that help lubricate the internal body, keeps you hydrated, reduces hunger, which helps with weight loss, and helps to make skin look smooth and young.

If you are not used to drinking water, it may seem hard at first, but very quickly, you will enjoy the clean, refreshed way it makes you feel. At a minimum, you should drink 64-ounces a day and more if you can.

For instance you may begin with 20 minutes every other day... then break those 20 minutes into smaller 'mini-intervals' as you get into better shape.

Shorter episodes will help you keep your muscle. When I'm teaching my anatomy and physiology classes at Barry University, I emphasize that muscles do more than facilitate movement. Your muscle mass is interconnected to your metabolism in the following ways:

- Fights fatigue, illness, sagging skin and bone fractures.

- Helps maintain a proper glucose balance.

- Increases your metabolic rate, reducing fat gain.

- Strengthens your immune system to decrease disease risk.

- To perform daily activities necessary for an independent quality lifestyle.

- Stores glycogen, which provides energy for the body.

This never-ending need for muscle continues throughout your life... especially as you reach your 60's, 70's and beyond. People with greater muscle mass benefit from proficient mental functioning, fewer chronic illnesses and a longer, healthier life.

Learn to Use Progressivity: The First Principle of PACE®

Many of my patients tell me they've been doing the same exercise for years without seeing results. And I'm not surprised... Aside from the problems with traditional "cardio" I mentioned in chapters 1 and 2, they have another common problem: *Endless Repetition*.

For any exercise program to continue to work through

Doctor's Tip:

Change your routine! Don't practice the same PACE routine for more than 6 to 8 weeks. By changing it up, you allow your body to make new adaptive responses. As your body responds to new challenges, you'll burn fat, and give your heart and lungs the reserve capacity they need to fight disease and prevent heart attacks.

time you must change something about the program. This is what I call progressivity and it is the first principle of your PACE® program. If you go to the gym and do the same routine for weeks, months and even years, you'll never make progress. Once your body makes an adaptive response to a fixed routine, <u>you need to change your routine</u>.

Doing the same workout repeatedly is the number one reason why people fail to make progress when they workout. This 10-minute workout is a good place to start, but if you do it for months without change, it will simply stop working. It will lose its effectiveness and you'll lose the progress you achieved.

As you read through the rest of this book, keep that in mind. In chapter 5, I'll give you new routines that build on this one. As you become more familiar with PACE®, you'll start to recognize the progressive element.

And it's this progressive feature that will continue to keep you fat-free – and disease-free – for life.

Get *Progressive* with Your First PACE® Workout

Now that you've had some experience with your 10-minute workout, go back and do it again. This time, you're going to add a ***progressive element***. Progressivity means making small changes in the same direction.

This is a critical element of PACE®, as it enables your body to make new adaptive responses. And these adaptive responses trigger all the benefits.

Let's say you did your 10-minute workout on a stationary bike three times a week for two weeks. And let's say you had your resistance set to "3." Of course, depending on what brand of stationary bike you're using, the settings will be different. But for the sake of argument, let's say that resistance level "1" is the lowest and "10" is the highest.

To make progressive changes, move your resistance level to "4" or "5" depending on how you feel. This will make it harder to pedal and will increase your challenge. Instead of doing 60-second exertion periods, <u>decrease them to 50 seconds</u>.

Try this new challenge for another two weeks.

Progressivity in Action: The Twin Study

In 2005, my **Wellness Research Foundation** conducted one of the most exciting clinical studies I've ever been involved with. We put PACE® to the test by studying two identical twins.

When they arrived for their initial assessment, both twins – age 18 – had identical body composition measurements. (Body composition measures the amount of body fat and lean body mass, or muscle.)

At the start of the study, both twins ran one mile each, three times a week. Over the course of 16 weeks, the "PACE" twin progressively decreased her distance to fit the PACE® program. The "cardio" twin progressively increased her distance to match a traditional cardio routine.

By the end of the study, the PACE® twin was *sprinting* 6 exercise sets. Each set had a 50-yard exertion interval followed by a recovery period of 30 seconds. The cardio twin was *jogging* 10 miles straight with no breaks.

The results? The PACE® twin went from 24.5% body fat all the way down to 10% for a total fat loss of 18 pounds. What's more, she gained 9 pounds of pure muscle.

The cardio twin lost fat, but not as much. She also started

at 24.5% body fat but went down to only 19.5% body fat for a total fat loss of 8 pounds. Not bad, but instead of gaining valuable muscle, the cardio twin actually lost 2 pounds of muscle.

Here's a look at their stats:

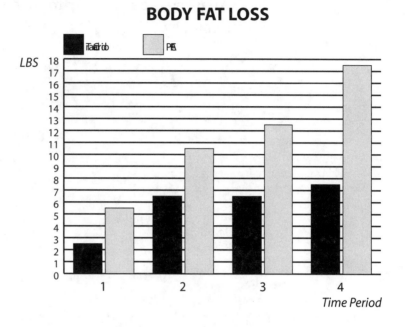

BODY FAT LOSS

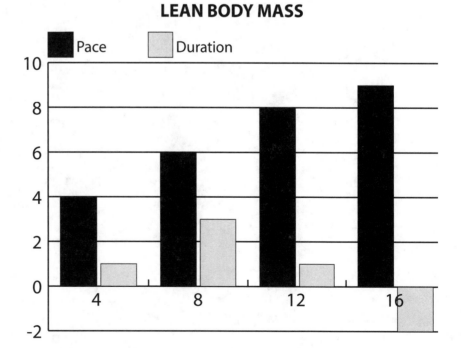

LEAN BODY MASS

Overall, **the PACE twin lost 125% more fat** than the cardio twin, and gained 9 pounds of muscle, where the cardio twin *lost muscle*.

And that's just the beginning... As you'll see later, some of my patients have experienced even more profound results. All using the same easy-to-follow principles you're learning right now.

CHAPTER 4
Set Your PACE® on Track

Y ou can use PACE® to change both your metabolism and your anatomy for the better. <u>This means less fat and more muscle</u>.

Now that you have a simple PACE® program to get you started, you need some additional tools to make your program effective. Good visualization is often the key to doing good work. Just as a carpenter needs good light at his workbench, you need to illuminate your starting points if you want to change your metabolism and your anatomy.

PACE® will change your anatomy by reducing your body fat, especially if you are starting with excessive body fat. And in contrast to continuous duration "cardio," which burns off your muscle, PACE® will **build** muscle. And unlike aerobic exercise, which shrinks your lungs, exercising in your <u>supra-aerobic zone</u> will **expand** your lungs.

You will find PACE® to be a very effective tool to rapidly change certain aspects of your physiology or metabolism. When you challenge your body's capacity to produce high-energy output, <u>your body responds by storing more high-energy fuel</u>.

When you ask you heart rate to respond to high output, your body gets better at responding by adjusting the physiology that controls your heart rate. Just as we do in our clinic, you can take measurements to track these changes.

You will use 2 simple measurements as tools for progress. These tools will help you discover your starting point, measure your changes, keep you on track and verify your benefits as you progress through PACE®.

Let's start with measuring your anatomy. Since you will be using PACE® to get and stay lean, we need a measurement to track your body fat.

Are You Fit or Fat?

It's a simple matter to measure the difference between fit and fat. However, you need to know that all obesity statistics use an outdated system called the BMI or Body Mass Index. It's a calculation based on height and weight. But it doesn't differentiate fat from muscle.

Because it is nonspecific and means almost nothing, forget about BMI and scale weight completely.

Since muscle is denser than fat, it will increase your BMI score more than fat will. And this failure exposes the BMI measurement to a huge potential for error. My own BMI calculates to 29. This would lead you to believe that I am overweight, almost obese. Yet, I have only 12% body fat.

Under the BMI system, people with a lot of muscle will have a higher score and will be considered "overweight" (BMI score of 25 to 29.9) or "obese," (BMI score above 30) even though they may be extremely fit.

According to the BMI, these celebrities are "overweight":

Celebrity	Height	Weight	BMI Score
Michael Jordan	6' 6"	216	25
Will Smith	6' 2"	210	27
George Clooney	5' 11"	211	29

I bet these Hollywood insiders never realized they were "obese."

Celebrity	Height	Weight	BMI Score
Mel Gibson	5' 9"	214	32
Arnold Schwarzenegger	6' 2"	257	33
Sylvester Stallone	5' 9"	228	34

So what is the solution to finding your meaningful measurement for how fit or fat you are?

Use your **body composition**. This measures how much of your weight is fat and how much is lean muscle mass. Men should have 10-20% body fat and women should have 15-25%. There is little point in measuring more than once every two weeks. Once a month is usually enough for most people.

As you focus on your fitness goals, aim to <u>increase lean body mass and reduce body fat</u>.

The ratio of fat to lean body mass is the real measurement of health. To go back to our twin study from the last chapter, here's the **body composition** of the "PACE" twin who lost 18 pounds of fat and gained 9 pounds of muscle over 16 weeks.

You don't need a complicated BMI chart or graph – any of the three following methods will measure your body composition:

Date	Apr 7, 2005	Apr 28, 2005	May 19, 2005	June 2, 2005	Aug 18, 2005
Weight	118	116	113	113	109
% of Body Fat	24.5	19.5	16.3	14.2	10
Lbs. of Fat	29	23	18	16	11
Lbs. of Lean Body Mass	89	93	95	97	98

1. **Electrical Impedance** – This is not the most accurate testing method (calipers are better), but this simply requires you to step on a scale and enter a few numbers. This method uses your body's conductivity to calculate your body fat, since water-based tissues are good electrical conductors and fats are insulators. The scale makes the calculations for you.

This measurement tracks changes if you measure at the same time of day, although they can still be inaccurate. K-Mart and Wal-Mart stores carry a popular brand of these scales.

2. **Circumference Measurement** – This is another simple, but not necessarily easy, way to measure your waist and hip girths. Wrap a tape measure around your waist at your navel and record the number of inches. Then, measure your hips at their widest point. Your goal is to have your waist measure at least 1 inch less than your hips (for both men and women). (www.accufitness.com)

3. **Skin Fold Test** – This is the most accurate and easiest way to measure your body composition. Using skin calipers, you measure skin folds to determine the percentage of body fat. In less than 5 minutes, you can get a correct measurement. (www.alsearsmd.com/catalog)

Your Heart Rate: The Key to Effective Exercise

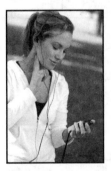

Your pulse rate – the speedometer of your heart – is the number of times your heart beats per minute. Your pulse tells you how fast you're going and whether you need to speed up or slow down – depending on your optimal conditioning zone.

You can measure your heart rate at two

pulse points: inside the wrist and the carotid artery in the neck. (The carotid artery carries blood to your brain and can be found by running your index and middle fingers along your windpipe.)

You will use 3 measurements to approximate your heart health and track your PACE® progress:

- Resting Heart Rate

- Maximum Heart Rate Achieved During Exertion

- Recovery Heart Rate

Generally, the lower your pulse rate, the fitter you are – unless you have a pacemaker or heart disease. Your pulse rises to meet the demands of an activity and then recovers when you rest.

Your heart's rate when you're at rest is your **resting heart rate**. As you start to exercise, your heart rate speeds up. The "top speed" your heart achieves at the peak of your exercise routine is your **maximum heart rate achieved**.

The time it takes for your pulse to go from its exercise rate down to its resting rate is called your **recovery time**. And your heart rate after you've stopped exercising for a few minutes is your **recovery heart rate**.

As you get into better shape, your resting pulse rate will be lower and your speed of recovery will increase.

What is *Your* Heart Rate?

The average *resting* heart rate for an adult is between 60 and 100 beats per minute. Well-conditioned athletes can have a resting pulse between 40 and 60 beats per minute.

Resting Pulse – To determine your pulse rate do the following:

- Sit quietly for two minutes and then find your pulse.

- Count the number of beats you feel in ten seconds.

- Write down that number and multiply by six.

- Repeat this process two more times and record your results.

- Calculate the average (mean) of these three results.

- **This is your Resting Pulse**.

Determing Your Resting Pulse Rate
Number of beats in 10 seconds (1st time) × 6 = _____
Number of beats in 10 seconds (2nd time) × 6 = _____
Number of beats in 10 seconds (3rd time) × 6 = _____
Total Beats ÷ 3 = _____ **Resting Pulse Rate**

Find Your Maximum Heart Rate for a Safe and Effective PACE® Workout

Your **maximum heart rate** and your **maximum heart rate achieved during exertion** are <u>two different measurements</u>.

Your **maximum heart rate** is simply a guideline. It represents a range you should aim for during exercise.

Your **maximum heart rate achieved during exercise** is the actual number you reach during your workout. This will change from day to day. I'll tell you how to measure that in just a minute. First, let's find the range for your maximum heart rate.

Your **maximum heart rate** is 220 minus your age. <u>The target for a healthy pulse rate during or immediately following exercise is 60 to 80 percent of this number</u>. If you're 50 years old, you subtract 50 from 220 to get 170. Sixty percent of 170 is 102. That's the bottom of your range. Eighty percent of 170 is 136. That's the top of your range.

- If you are age 50, you should aim to build up your fitness level gradually, until you reach a target pulse rate during exercise between 102-136 bpm, (beats per minute).

- Age 55, your target should be between 99-132 bpm.

- Age 60, your target should be between 96-128 bpm.

- Age 65, your target should be between 93-124 bpm.

- Age 70, your target should be between 90-120 bpm.

- Age 75, your target should be between 87-116 bpm.

These target rates are only guidelines, as your pulse rate may be affected by other factors such as medication, pacemakers, or certain forms of heart disease. If any of these apply to you, your doctor will be able to set a target pulse rate for you.

Heart Rate Journal		
Date	Target Rate Range	Actual Rate
12/15	99-132	103

Sample Heart Rate Journal.
A chart for your use can be found in Appendix C.

Keep in mind that some variations may apply. If you're out of shape when you start, you'll need to make some adjustments. Some of my patients are so deconditioned; their hearts take 20 minutes just to recover from a brisk walk. On the other hand, I have a 65-year old patient who gets his heart rate up to 170 without much effort – far above the average for his age.

If your pulse is less than your target range during exercise, you can speed up or work harder. You'll need to slow down if your pulse rate is more than your target range. Most importantly, be sure to pace yourself to maximize ultimate benefits.

Keep track of the time it takes for your pulse rate – during exercise – to return to its normal resting rate after you exercise. Within four weeks of starting regular exercise, you'll see a noticeable reduction in *recovery time*.

As you'll see, recovery time is critical to the success of your PACE® program. It's a very clear and accurate measure of your progress. The faster your recovery time, the healthier your heart is. So if you're feeling out of shape, extend your *rest periods*. Make sure your heart rate recovers to its resting rate before you do another *exercise set*. As you progress, your recovery time will speed up.

Children often have very fast recovery times. Because their hearts are young and resilient, they can run around at break-neck speed and be back to normal in seconds.

A few years ago, when my son was 5 or 6 years old, I had him run around the pool as fast as he could. I then measured his heart rate. It was an extremely fast 240 beats per minute. I measured again only 15 seconds later. It had returned to 120!

You should consult your doctor if your heart rate does not come down within a few minutes of stopping exercise. Also see a doctor if you feel any of the following during exercise: an irregular or rapid heartbeat, light-headedness, dizziness, fainting, and shortness of breath or chest pain.

How Fast Does Your Heart Beat During Exercise?

Now you're going to find your exercise pulse, or your **maximum heart rate achieved during exercise**.

Exercise Pulse – To determine your Exercise Pulse, follow these directions:

1. Do 50 jumping jacks **without stopping**. When you finish, you should be out of breath.

2. Immediately sit down and find your pulse.

3. Count the number of beats in 10 seconds.

4. Now multiply by 6.

5. **This is your Exercise Pulse.**

Recovery Heart Rate: Your *True* Measure of Heart Health

A study in The New England Journal of Medicine shows that one of the best tests to predict your chance of dying in the near future is your **Recovery Heart Rate**. To measure your recovery heart rate, do the following:

1. Exercise steadily until you start breathing heavily.

2. Record your heart rate.

3. Hold that pace for at least a minute.

4. Cool down for two minutes.

5. Measure your pulse rate exactly one minute after stopping.

6. **This is your Recovery Heart Rate.**

Let's say you're on the treadmill and you start to breathe heavily. You measure your heart rate, and the result is 150. Keep going at that pace for another minute. Then start a cool down period where you slow down to walking speed. Do that for 2 minutes, then stop completely. Now measure your heart rate exactly 60 seconds after you stop. That's your recovery heart rate.

If your heart does not slow down at least 30 beats in the first minute, you are in poor shape and at increased risk for a heart attack. If your recovery heart rate slows down more than fifty beats in the first minute, you are in excellent shape.

Note: This test can cause irregular heartbeats in people with damaged hearts, so check with your physician before you try it.

Once you become familiar with these numbers, you can start to track your progress. Some people skip this part of the program, but I urge you not to. **If you don't monitor your progress, you won't make any!**

A few years ago, I had a patient – JF – who has very out of shape. I put her on the treadmill for just a few minutes at a low intensity. Within no time, she was ready to fall over. I told her to stop and rest. After a full 5 minutes of walking slowly, her heart was still beating at 140!

Doctor's Tip:

Exercising with a partner makes you accountable to someone else for each workout and can improve adherence to a program. A partner can inspire you to push yourself a little bit harder when your energy levels are not at its peak.

She was discouraged, but I told her not worry about her results. I made sure she kept a log of her workouts and then followed up with her week by week. What a difference! After 12 weeks, her heart was fully recovering from her exercise routine in just over a minute.

So keep a log and write everything down. Don't allow yourself to be discouraged. After a few weeks when your body adapts and your heart strengthens, you'll be glad you did.

CHAPTER 5

Advance Your PACE®
to the Next Level

Now that you've done your first PACE® routine and you've logged your starting points, you can add the elements that make PACE® uniquely effective.

In a nutshell, you'll use this system to practice and train your ability to use energy at a higher rate – this is your **high-energy output system** we talked about in chapter 2. And you'll practice and train getting to that higher output faster.

Why bother?

Because if you never challenge your current aerobic capacity, breathing rate, cardiac output or the maximal metabolic rate that you can achieve, these systems will inevitably decline – in the same way that muscles you don't challenge will weaken and atrophy.

If you've ever broken a bone and worn a cast, you know how fast and far muscles you're not using shrink. Your physiology and "metabolic fitness" adapt and respond in the same way.

The training of your high-energy output system is critical to your health improvement, disease resistance, fat-fighting, energizing and anti-aging capacities. It's incredible that no popular exercise program has ever specifically addressed this issue.

On the surface, it would be dangerous – even foolhardy – to go on an intense exercise rampage to challenge your heart, lung, vascular and metabolic capacities. What you need is a plan to build these capacities safely and effectively.

> **Doctor's Tip:**
>
> During sleep, your body is resting and recovering from all the work is has done throughout the day. Your serotonin levels are brought back in line, your muscles relax, and mind is allowed to clear itself in preparation for the next day. If you are not getting the proper amount of sleep, you will notice it in a physical way. Usually between six and eight hours a night is appropriate.

PACE® is the first and only program conceived, designed, tested and proven to achieve this most important of all fitness goals. It does this for you by measuring where you are, then making progressive, small, incremental changes over time.

It is a flexible plan that works equally well for athletic power lifters, marathoners, extremely deconditioned couch potatoes, overly aerobicized fitness buffs, elders and even heart patients in rehabilitation. It is effective and safe because of its flexibility.

It's flexible because it's not focused on what you do as much as the direction of your change over time.

The key is to start with a brief exertion that is comfortable for you at your current capacity. It's not so important how hard you exert yourself today. It's that little bit that you do next week that you didn't do this week.

That tiny incremental change compounds – like interest on capital – to have an amazing and powerful affect over time. By changing your program through time, you work with your metabolism and your inborn adaptive response to coach your body to change.

Accelerate Your PACE® Program to Boost Your Heart Rate and Lung Volume

Here's a real clinical example to illustrate: A male patient in his mid 30s – JH – came to me with 35% body fat. He was very out of shape and reported low energy, depression and some difficulty taking full, deep breaths.

His progress is a perfect example of not only fat burning, but of progressivity and *acceleration*. Acceleration simply means challenging your heart, lungs, blood vessels and your physiological and metabolic response a little faster.

Progressivity of the challenge will give you power in your response. Acceleration will give you speed in your response.

To help him make these changes, I created a program to help boost his heart rate and lung volume over time.

	Warm Up	Set 1		Set 2		Set 3	
Weeks		Exertion	Recovery	Exertion	Recovery	Exertion	Recovery
1 & 2	6 min **R2**	10 min	6 min				
3 & 4	5 min **R3**	8 min	4 min	8 min	4 min		
5 & 6	5 min **R4**	6 min	3 min	6 min	3 min	6 min	3 min
7 & 8	4 min **R4**	4 min	2 min	4 min **R5**	2 min	3 min	2 min
9 & 10	4 min **R4**	3 min	2 min	3 min **R5**	2 min	2 min **R6**	2 min
11 & 12	4 min **R4**	3 min	2 min	3 min **R5**	2 min	2 min **R6**	2 min
13 & 14	3 min **R5**	2 min	2 min	90 sec **R6**	2 min	1 min **R7**	2 min
15 & 16	3 min **R5**	2 min	2 min	90 sec **R6**	2 min	1 min **R7**	2 min
17 & 18	2 min **R5**	2 min	2 min	90 sec **R6**	2 min	1 min **R7**	2 min
19 & 20	1 min **R5**	2 min	2 min	90 sec **R6**	2 min	1 min **R7**	2 min

	Set 4		Set 5	
Weeks	Exertion	Recovery	Exertion	Recovery
1 & 2				
3 & 4				
5 & 6				
7 & 8				
9 & 10				
11 & 12	1 min **R7**	2 min		
13 & 14	1 min **R8**	2 min		
15 & 16	40 sec **R8**	2 min	30 sec **R8**	2 min
17 & 18	40 sec **R8**	2 min	30 sec **R9**	2 min
19 & 20	40 sec **R8**	2 min	30 sec **R9**	2 min

(I've created a blank chart just like this for you to use. You'll find it in Appendix C.)

Notice the ***progressively accelerating*** qualities of this workout. Over time, ***exercise sets*** are added – up to 5 by the 15th week. In addition, the **duration** of each exertion period decreases over time.

For this example, I've included the resistance settings in **bold**. (**R2**, **R3**, etc.) This will help you see how the challenge was increased over time. For weeks 1 & 2, the resistance level is set at only 2, which is a very mild challenge. But by week 17 and beyond, the 5th exertion period has a resistance level of 9, which creates a very intense, very challenging 30-second workout.

There's another aspect of *acceleration* that I want to point out here – something that you can't see on a chart: How quickly you challenge your heart and lungs during each exertion period.

Let's say your exertion period is 3 minutes and your resistance level is 4. When you begin that exertion period, you'll start at a moderate pace. After 20 to 30 seconds you'll feel your heart beat faster and your breathing become heavier. After about a minute, you'll hit your stride and carry on at the same pace until your 3 minutes is up.

But as you become more conditioned, you'll accelerate faster during each exertion period. Instead of taking 20 to 30 seconds to feel your heart and lungs adapt, your body will react faster. You'll hit your stride sooner, and carry it longer.

By the time you work up to 30-second exertion periods, the quality of your acceleration will enable you to hit the ground running.

After 20 weeks, JH went from 35% body fat down to just 18%. Take a look at his stats:

Date	5/10/05	6/16/05	7/12/05	8/03/05	9/02/05	10/11/05
Weight	166	169	176	178	170	170
% of Body Fat	35	33.3	29	27	22	18
Lbs. of Fat	58	56	51	48	37	31
Lbs. of Lean Body Mass	108	113	125	130	133	139
Max Heart Rate	144	149	151	158	163	170

Aside from his fat loss, the progressively accelerating quality of his workout produced a remarkable increase in his maximum heart rate.

(Appendix C includes a blank chart for you to record your own information and track your progress.)

When he started, he was very out of shape and could not adapt to the increase in cardiac demand. **But over time, his heart and lungs adapted *faster* to each new challenge.** The result is a stronger, more resilient heart with greater reserve capacity.

He also reported increased lung capacity, saying that for the first time in his life he could fully expand his lungs – especially in his upper chest – and take a deep breath.

The 4-Week Progression: Your Easy 12-Minute PACE® Program

Here's a simple program to use progressivity in the right direction. In the following 12-minute program, you're going to focus on gradually increasing the challenge as you progress.

To aid in this effort, and to make your body accept the proper signal to gear up your metabolism, this program also simultaneously decreases the duration of the exercise period. This has synergistic power that will surprise you.

Week	Warm Up	Set 1		Set 2		Set 3	
		Exertion	Recovery	Exertion	Recovery	Exertion	Recovery
1	3 min	6 min	3 min				
2	2 min	3 min	2 min	3 min	2 min		
3	2 min	2 min	2 min	2 min	2 min	2 min	2 min
4	3 min	1 min	2 min	1 min	2 min	1 min	2 min

You'll find a blank copy of this chart in Appendix C.

Remember don't stress yourself. It's not necessary to work that intensely. <u>By decreasing the duration, it will actually feel easier as the 4 weeks progress.</u>

Yet by the end of just 4 weeks, you will have changed from one set of 6 minutes of moderate exertion to 3 sets of just a slightly higher level of exertion. This progressivity in the right direction toward maximal capacity is the heart of PACE˙.

During week 1, you're going to take it easy and just do one warm up for 3 minutes and then one exercise set at a <u>low to moderate</u> intensity. Just do what feels comfortable. If you are not in very good shape, just start with walking.

Go slow for the warm-up, pick up the pace of your walk a little during the exertion period and drop to a slow pace again during the recovery. During each recovery period focus on returning you breathing rate to near your resting rate – about 12 to 16 breaths per minute is ideal.

Try and do this 20-minute interval at least 3 times during the first week. <u>But each time you do it, slightly increase the intensity level</u>. By the end of the first week, you should feel like you've given yourself a slight challenge you were able to accomplish.

Note: How you adjust the intensity, will depend on what instrument you're using. If you're on a stationary bike, increase the level on the control panel so it becomes harder to pedal. If you're on an elliptical, boost the incline so it's harder to run, etc.

How hard you push yourself should depend on your current level of conditioning. At this beginning stage, don't push yourself too hard. This is just a warm-up.

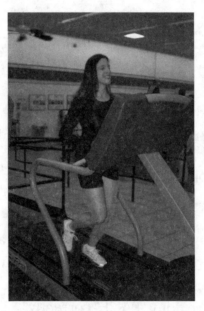

During week 2, you'll add another exercise set. But the duration of your exertion periods will decrease. After a 2-minute warm up, you'll do a 3-minute exertion period. As you start, notice how fast you're going and how long it takes for your heart and lungs to meet the challenge.

When 3 minutes is up, begin your recovery. If you need to stop, that's okay. Otherwise, your recovery period should be a slow, easy pace. If you're on an elliptical machine for example, you should slow down so you feel like you're walking.

As always during your recovery period, focus on your heart rate slowing down. If you start to pant, let it happen. Feel your lungs quickly fill up and release. Allow your body to come back to a state of rest.

During week 3, you'll start with a 2-minute warm up and then a 2-minute exertion period. <u>But this time, increase the intensity to give yourself more of a challenge</u>.

When 2 minutes is up, begin your recovery. Repeat this process for exercise sets 2 and 3. During week 3, try and repeat this workout 3 or 4 times.

When you hit week 4, you're going to do 3 exercise sets as in week 3. Except this time, you're going to reduce the exertion periods to just 1 minute each, followed by 2-minute recovery periods.

Apply the same principles. Take your warm up at a low to moderate intensity. Then turn up the intensity when you start your first exertion period.

Get the Most Out of Your PACE® Workout – Use a Heart Rate Monitor

The advantage of working out in the gym is the easy access to heart rate monitors. Most machines have them built in.

(Personal heart rate monitors are available through: www.accufitness.com)

Remember in chapter 2 we talked about something called an oxygen deficit? As you start your PACE® program, try and get a feel for what this is. It's a sure-fire way of knowing if you're doing PACE® correctly.

How do you know if you're creating an oxygen deficit? Easy... **Look at your heart rate monitor**. When you finish an exertion period and go into a recovery period, your heart rate should go up a few ticks. This usually takes place in the first 10 to 15 seconds. As your recovery period continues, then your heart rate will start to come down.

Here's a quick example of what I mean: Let's say you're coming to the end of your exertion period and you notice your heart rate is 155. When you finish your exertion period, you'll immediately slow down and begin your recovery. During this transition, your heart rate will actually go up a few points – and then begin to drop.

It's natural to think that your heart rate would immediately drop once you stop your exertion period and slow down. But when you've created an oxygen debt, your heart actually pumps faster for a few moments. You'll notice this if you're watching your heart rate monitor. This slight increase helps your heart deliver more oxygen to relieve the oxygen debt you created.

The second indicator is your breath. When you create an oxygen deficit, you start to pant and feel winded. This means you're asking your lungs to provide your body with more oxygen than it's able to supply at that given moment. As a result, you start to pant – making you breathe faster in an attempt to get more oxygen to you cells more quickly.

Congratulations! This means you've entered your *supra-aerobic zone*. Again, you'll feel the panting immediately after you finish your exertion period and drop into your recovery period. This is when you'll notice a brief increase in your heart rate.

These 2 indicators are signs that you're entering your *supra-aerobic zone*. Use them to your advantage!

Take Your PACE® Workout to the Next Level!

Once you get comfortable with the basics of PACE®, you'll be able to take on greater challenges. I've included some additional PACE® routines on the next page. These programs will speed your progress, as it's important to change your PACE® routine every 6 to 8 weeks.

PACE® 8-Week Intermediate Program

With this 8-week plan, you'll incorporate all the fundamentals of PACE®: intensity, acceleration, progressivity and decreasing duration. There are blank charts in Appendix C for you to fill in your own information.

Weeks	Warm Up	Set 1		Set 2		Set 3		Set 4	
		Exert.	Rec.	Exert.	Rec.	Exert.	Rec.	Exert.	Rec.
1 & 2	3 min	2 min	2 min	2 min	2 min	2 min	2 min	2 min	2 min
3 & 4	3 min	90 sec	2 min	90 sec	2 min	90 sec	2 min	90 sec	2 min
5 & 6	2 min	60 sec	2 min	60 sec	2 min	60 sec	2 min	60 sec	2 min
7 & 8	2 min	40 sec	2 min	40 sec	2 min	40 sec	2 min	40 sec	2 min

During your first 2 weeks, your exertion periods are the same length as your rest intervals. After you finish week 1, slightly <u>increase the intensity</u> of your exertion.

When you hit weeks 3 and 4, you'll <u>shorten the duration</u> of each exertion period but slightly <u>increase the intensity</u> further.

Doctor's Tip:

Find some time away from noise and distractions for you. Meditation can come in many forms. Whatever way you meditate, ensure that you are in a quiet place with soft lighting, sit with good posture and in a comfortable position, practice slow, rhythmic breathing, and concentrate on something calm and relaxing. Meditation is a great stress reducer, which is vital for good health.

At week 5, the pace continues to accelerate as your exertion period drops to 60 seconds. You'll notice that the rest interval remains the same throughout the 8 weeks. Use the recovery period to measure your recovery time.

As you move through this program, you should notice your recovery time improving. In other words, every time you move into a recovery period, you'll get back to your resting pulse more quickly.

By the time you get to weeks 7 and 8, your exertion period is just 40 seconds. During these periods, you should turn up the intensity even further and really give yourself a workout. When you get to a recovery period, you should be panting and out of breath.

The 5-Set, Short-Duration, High-Intensity Workout

This workout stands on its own. With these brief exertions you don't need to change their duration each week like the previous examples.

Warm Up	Set 1		Set 2		Set 3		Set 4		Set 5	
	Exert.	Rec.	Exert.	Rec.	Exert.	Rec.	Exert.	Rec.	Exert.	Rec.
90 sec	1 min	90 sec	50 sec	90 sec	40 sec	90 sec	30 sec	90 sec	20 sec	90 sec

A blank chart in Appendix C will help you keep track of your personal workout.

With this format, you should turn up the intensity after each interval. By the time you get to the 20-second exertion period, you should be giving it everything you have.

20 seconds of high-intensity exercise doesn't sound like much, but if you're doing right, you should be winded and gasping for air – and drenched in sweat! (Don't attempt this routine unless you've already gone through the previous programs.)

After a few weeks, apply the principle of progressivity and make some changes. First, you can try changing instruments. If you're using a stationary bike, switch to an elliptical. If you're already using the elliptical, switch to a recumbent bike, etc. (See chapter 7 for more on using different instruments.)

Doctor's Tip:

More intense workouts performed less often will actually produce greater results. Your body needs rest to recover and repair damaged muscle tissue and avoid injury.

When you feel you've reached a plateau, continue to make changes. Make your first exertion period 50 seconds instead of 60. Then change the next four exertion periods accordingly. But remember to turn up the intensity whenever you decrease the duration of an exertion period.

By now, you should have an intuitive sense of just how flexible the PACE® program really is.

Take it to the Max: Extreme PACE®

Okay... here's a workout for you die-hards. The ones who like to take things to the extreme. For this program, I suggest that you run – either on a treadmill or outside.

This program stretches out over five days. And you should focus on trying to <u>increase the intensity after each day</u>. A blank chart in Appendix C will help you track your progress.

After a quick look, you'll notice that days 1 to 3 have exertion periods measured in **distance**. Whereas days 4 and 5 are measured in **time**. The 100-yard exertion periods in day 3 should be treated as a "hundred-yard dash," that will set you up for the 15-second exertion periods in day 5, which should be seen as **sprints**.

This is a real challenge, so take it easy. If it gets to be too much, give it a rest and try it again another day. **Note:** 1/4 mile = 440 yards; 1/8 mile = 220 yards.

Day 1	Set 1		Set 2		Set 3	
Warm-up	Exertion	Recovery	Exertion	Recovery	Exertion	Recovery
2 min	1/4 mile	3 min	1/4 mile	3 min	1/4 mile	3 min

	Set 4		Set 5		Set 6	
	Exertion	Recovery	Exertion	Recovery	Exertion	Recovery
	1/8 mile	3 min	1/8 mile	3 min	1/8 mile	3 min

Day 2	Set 1		Set 2		Set 3	
Warm-up	Exertion	Recovery	Exertion	Recovery	Exertion	Recovery
2 min	200 yards	3 min	200 yards	3 min	175 yards	3 min

	Set 4		Set 5		Set 6	
	Exertion	Recovery	Exertion	Recovery	Exertion	Recovery
	175 yards	3 min	150 yards	3 min	150 yards	3 min

Day 3	Set 1		Set 2		Set 3	
Warm-up	Exertion	Recovery	Exertion	Recovery	Exertion	Recovery
2 min	150 yards	3 min	150 yards	3 min	150 yards	3 min

	Set 4		Set 5		Set 6	
	Exertion	Recovery	Exertion	Recovery	Exertion	Recovery
	100 yards	3 min	100 yards	3 min	100 yards	3 min

Day 4	Set 1		Set 2		Set 3	
Warm-up	Exertion	Recovery	Exertion	Recovery	Exertion	Recovery
2 min	40 sec	2 min	40 sec	2 min	40 sec	2 min

	Set 4		Set 5		Set 6	
	Exertion	Recovery	Exertion	Recovery	Exertion	Recovery
	30 sec	2 min	30 sec	2 min	30 sec	2 min

Day 5	Set 1		Set 2		Set 3	
Warm-up	Exertion	Recovery	Exertion	Recovery	Exertion	Recovery
2 min	30 sec	2 min	30 sec	2 min	20 sec	2 min

	Set 4		Set 5		Set 6	
	Exertion	Recovery	Exertion	Recovery	Exertion	Recovery
	20 sec	2 min	15 sec	2 min	15 sec	2 min

The key to a good exercise plan is to enjoy what you are doing. By alternating various exercises, you'll lower your chance of injuries and keep your routine fun. The goal is to incorporate activities that give your lungs and heart a workout.

Elliptical machines, stair stepping, swimming, sprinting, and biking are all excellent choices, depending on your

Doctor's Tip:

Look for a school with a track if you are not a member of a gym. There you can do sprints, etc. Many communities have local pools. If yours doesn't, look for a YMCA, many of which do have a pool.

level of fitness. These activities provide the correct cardiopulmonary challenge that you can control. I'll give you more tips and advice about different instruments in chapter 7.

To achieve maximum benefits, you should always do the following before beginning any exercise program:

- Do a light "warm up" and stretch before each session.

- Reduce muscle soreness after each session with a few minutes of a light "cool down."

- Clear your exercise program with your physician.

Keep in mind that PACE® should be adapted to *your* needs. If you're interested in the workouts you see in this book, but feel they're too intense – or not challenging enough – go ahead and play around with them. Take the initiative and improvise.

It's not the length of the exertion periods that makes PACE® worthwhile. It's your willingness to apply yourself, make changes over time and stick with your program.

CHAPTER 6

Build Strength the
Old–Fashioned Way

If you want real strength that you can use, forget lifting weights. If you just want larger muscles, then weight training is your best tool. If done properly, it will cause your muscle to enlarge.

But after all these years as a personal trainer, coach, fitness consultant and anti-aging physician I cannot escape one very negative limitation of weight training – you're not really training anything. What you're actually doing is conditioning your muscles to tense up, tearing fibers and creating bloated hypertrophied muscle fibers in response.

This new muscle mass becomes dysfunctional because it has become disconnected with central nervous system control of muscle's primary purpose – to move your body. It creates strength, tension and size imbalances, unnatural patterns of movement, malpositioned joints and sets you up for injuries. And it's certainly not the best way to build functional strength you can use.

Functional strength is what enables you to climb flights of stairs while you're carrying 4 bags of groceries without injuring yourself. It propels you out of bed in the morning and helps you carry out life's daily tasks. And as you get older, it's keeping your functional strength that will keep you mobile, independent and out of the nursing home until the day you arrive at the Pearly Gates.

What's more, your body is not designed for the mechanics of weight lifting patterns. For someone with low muscle mass a well designed lower body resistance workout can help restore the lost mass. But for many in my clinics, the recurrent unnatural strain has produced way too many injuries.

Other research shows that blood pressure can spike as high as 370/360 during a lift. (Normal resting blood pressure is below 130/80.) And, aside from causing frequent joint, muscle and tendon overuse injuries, weight lifting can lead to high blood pressure, aneurysms, strokes, even a fatal arterial disease known as dissection – especially in older folks.[1]

Nature designed your body to build and maintain muscle in response to the demands of **your own body weight**. "Exercising" this natural function, i.e. – moving your body weight – is also the most effective way to strengthen ligaments and tendons.

Before the modern fads of aerobics, cardio and weight lifting took over and created the commercialized modern gyms, going to the gym used to mean boxing, wrestling, pushups, chin-ups and calisthenics.

After trying it all myself and testing and researching strength building for 30 years, the best way to build the kind of functional strength that you use in normal daily activities remains good old-fashioned *calisthenics*.

The Greek word "calisthenics" comes from 'kallos' for beauty and 'thenos' for strength.[2] One minor warning- these exercises are often harder than they look. But practiced over time, they make it easier to perform routine physical tasks, and they improve bone density, metabolism and immune function. They are also at the core of the strength-training program for the U.S. Green Berets and Navy Seals.

You can do calisthenics whether you're on the road, in the office, or at home. It's the perfect "any time, anywhere" exercise. No special or expensive equipment is necessary and with a few simple maneuvers, you can exercise multiple muscle groups.

As with any exercise program, begin slowly. In just a few weeks, you should see results, if you remain consistent and stay with the program. You'll need to build up your stamina by starting slowly and increasing your endurance.

Get the 8 Benefits of Strong Muscles

Here are the top 8 benefits of a strength-training program:[3]

1. Lower resting blood pressure.
2. Reduction of body fat.
3. Reduction of symptoms associated with Type II diabetes: depression, sleep disorders, osteoporosis and depression.
4. Muscle strength is increased and muscle loss is prevented.
5. Increased bone mass and density to protect against osteoporosis, (a disease that affects bone fragility).
6. Alleviates lower back pain and increases lower back strength.
7. Improves functional flexibility and strength, keeping you safe during daily activities.
8. Improves personal appearance, physique, self-esteem and self-confidence.

Calisthenics Speed Your Recovery from Heart Disease

People of all ages benefit from muscular conditioning, especially those needing to recover from heart disease.

As we get older, muscle wasting causes us to lose the ability to move our bodies, often requiring the assistance of walking aids and wheelchairs. By increasing the size of your muscles, you also improve your stamina and stability.

Using a functional resistance-training program, such as calisthenics, is your best approach to muscle conditioning. Strengthening your muscle capacity creates positive muscle adaptation. This makes performing everyday physical activities less challenging.

Doctor's Tip:

When a person gets a therapeutic massage, they are actually getting the benefit of function improvement with circulatory, muscular, skeletal, nervous systems, lymphatic, and can even help the body heal after an illness or injury.

I like to begin with several repetitions of arm circles, leg lifts, upper body rotations, and hurdle steps. Moving your body through these physical motions will prevent injury by loosening joints and tendons.

Lower Body Strength: Your Key to Life-Long Mobility

Your lower body is more important for functional strength than your upper body. These muscles are bigger and meant to be stronger. They provide your foundation and you should focus on strengthening them first.

Your three biggest muscles work to flex and extend your hip joint. These muscles are:

- Quadriceps on the front of your thighs.

- Hamstrings on the back of your thighs.

- Gluteus muscles in your buttocks.

Four of the best exercises for these muscles are:

- **Hindu Squats** – Stand with your feet shoulder width apart. Extend your arms out in front of you, parallel to the ground with your hands open and palms facing down. Inhale briskly and pull your hands straight back. As you pull back, turn the wrists up and make a fist. At the end of the inhalation, your elbows should be behind you with both hands in a fist, palm side up.

  From this position, exhale, bend your knees and squat. Let your arms fall to your sides and touch ground with the tips of your fingers. Continue exhaling and let your arms swing up as you stand.

  This brings you back to the starting position: standing straight up with your arms extended in front of you, hands open and palms facing down.

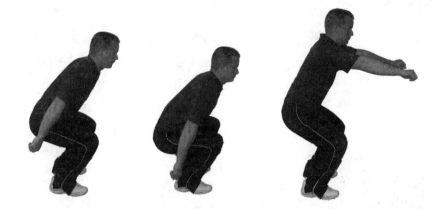

Repeat at the pace of one repetition every four seconds. Once you are comfortable with the form, you can increase your speed to one squat per second.

Repeat until you feel winded. Rest, recover and do another set. Once you're conditioned, you'll be able to do one hundred repetitions in a set. (I do five hundred every other day…) *Many thanks to my friend Matt Furey for teaching me this exercise.*

• **Alternating Lunges** - With your hands on your hips, take a step forward with your right leg until your front knee is bent 90 degrees and your back knee almost touches the ground. Push off from your leading foot and return to the starting position. Repeat with your left leg.

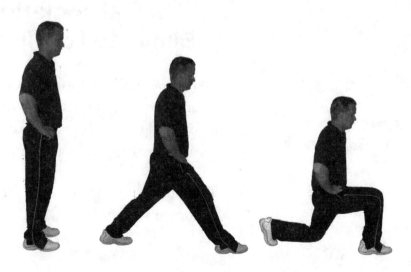

- **Squats** – With feet shoulder width apart, squat as far as possible. Bring your arms forward, parallel to the floor. Return to standing position. Repeat.

- **Jump Squats** – With body crouched, feet together, arms at sides, head straight and level, quickly straighten legs and jump upward as high as you can. Simultaneously, extend arms and reach overhead. After landing, quickly return to original position, without losing your balance. Repeat.

Begin with these muscles and work them first if you want to maximize the effect on your total body strength.[4]

Get Rock-Hard Abs and Eliminate Pain in Your Lower Back

To prevent pain and injury in the lower back, you must have strong abdominal muscles. Functional strength is supported by building powerful core muscle groups to improve your breath, posture, and mechanics of motion.

The four best floor exercises for concentrating on your abdomen include:

- **Crunches/Sit-Ups** – Lie on your back, raise your head slightly, hold, and repeat.

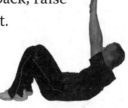

- **Leg Levers** – Lie on your back, legs six inches off the ground. Lift legs another foot higher, return to starting position. Repeat.

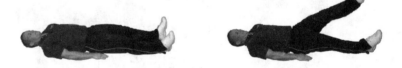

- **Back Flutter Kicks** – Lie on your back, and alternate each leg 2 to 3 feet off ground. Repeat.

- **Scissors** – Lie on your back, raise legs a few inches off ground. Spread legs apart and then bring them together. Repeat.

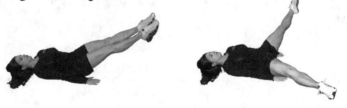

Pump Up Your Upper Body Strength
Without Going to the Gym

You build practical strength by engaging in a full-range of motion activities. Challenge your upper body by using your own body weight. Everyday activities, like lifting heavy packages or moving furniture, will be easier as your muscles build useful strength.

To prevent injury, focus more on your back than your chest and arms. The best exercises for building upper body strength include:

- **Pushups** – Lie face down. Place hands a little wider than shoulder-width apart. Straighten your back and place feet together. Lower yourself until you almost touch the ground. (Keep knees on the ground and feet in the air if this is too difficult.)

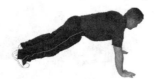 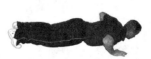

- **Pull-Ups** – Palms face out for a traditional pull-up on bar to strengthen middle back muscles. Palms face toward you to do a chin-up, which strengthens the back and biceps.

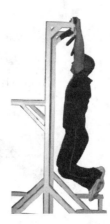 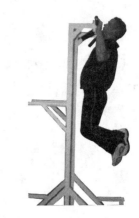

- **Dips** – Use parallel bars, two chairs or two desks. Put feet on the ground, while putting one hand on each object. Slowly lower yourself until elbows are at 90-degree angles. Pause. Slowly raise yourself. Repeat. Excellent exercise for chest, middle back and triceps.

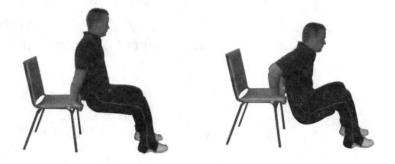

- **Arm Haulers** – Lie on your stomach. Stretch your arms in front of you. Raise arms and legs off floor and sweep arms back to your thighs (similar to a breaststroke.) Return arms to starting position. Repeat.

You can alternate with these other bodyweight exercises:

- **Instep Touches** – Stand with feet shoulder-width apart, toes slightly pointing outwards, arms extended to your sides and parallel to the floor, head straight and level. Bend forward at your waist, turn your upper body, and bring the fingers of one hand to instep of opposite foot. Keep arms and legs straight but not locked. Simultaneously, raise your other arm to ceiling. Repeat.

- **Knee Bends** – With feet almost together and arms at sides, head straight and level, bend your knees to lower your body. When thighs are parallel, rise up on your toes, while simultaneously swinging your arms forward. Your arms will be parallel to the floor in front of you, with fingers together and palms facing down and back, remaining perpendicular to the floor.

Reverse this motion, without stopping, and return to original starting position. Repeat.

If you feel any dizziness, shortness of breath or pain, slow down. Do not over-exert yourself. If done effectively, you will transform your body through the power of calisthenics. By doing a regular calisthenics routine, you'll see improvements in your stamina and appearance.

P ACE® is so versatile; you can use it with any machine, instrument, sport or activity that can give your heart and lungs a challenge. While running and biking are the most common, you have a wide variety of options to help you achieve your fitness goals.

Here's my top 12 list, with a few words of advice for each:

1. Outdoor Sprints/Running: This is my personal favorite. I practice PACE® on dirt roads around my house in the early morning. If possible, find a quiet area, with a pleasing ambiance that doesn't get a lot of traffic. Inside a park is usually good.

One of the benefits of outdoor running is variation. You can practice exertion based on either time or distance. Timed periods are great for gradually decreasing the duration of your exertion periods. As you gradually decrease the time of exertion in each set, you'll find it easier to really work on creating an oxygen debt and panting during your recovery. This is great for developing lungpower and burning fat in the "afterburn" after your exercise.

> **Doctor's Tip:**
>
> Your body was created with a built in cooling system, called sweat or if you prefer, perspiration. Sweat is a vital key in a good workout. When your body heats up do to exertion, sweat is doing the job intended – keeping the body cool.

If you are measuring your distance, you can practice PACE® without timing yourself. For each exertion period you can run a preset distance like the length of your block. For each recovery, you can walk the same distance back to your starting point. Then, over several weeks with this routine, you can keep the distance in each set the same while you gradually increase the number of sets as you become more conditioned. This is great for burning off calories while you preserve your reserve capacity in your heart.

Keep in mind that outdoor running in brief gradually changing periods of exertion has quite a different affect on your metabolism than jogging. Don't let the "runners high" fool you. The reason distance runners get that feeling is that they secrete endorphins, your body's opiate-like pain relievers. Why does your body release these morphine like substance in your brain? To get you through the stress.

Your body interprets longer duration cardio as stress. Some people learn to like the high but over the long run, the stress inevitably will take its toll. Yet outdoor running in brief exertion sets actually becomes more rewarding the more you use PACE®.

For distance periods, if you like you can measure off sections of 50, 100 and 220 yards. For timed periods, having a circuit or circular area can make it easier but it's not necessary.

Outdoor Running: Distance

	Set 1		Set 2		Set 3	
Warm-up	Exertion	Recovery	Exertion	Recovery	Exertion	Recovery
2 min	1/8 mile	3 min	1/8 mile	3 min	100 yards	3 min

Set 4		Set 5		Set 6	
Exertion	Recovery	Exertion	Recovery	Exertion	Recovery
100 yards	3 min	50 yards	3 min	50 yards	3 min

If you are in good cardiovascular condition you can start your first exertion period by running an eighth of a mile (220 yards). Your intensity level should be low to moderate. After each recovery period, <u>increase the intensity</u>. By the time you reach your 6th exertion period, you should be **sprinting**.

If this is too tough, don't despair. If you get out of breath with 10 steps, it's OK. Rest while you focus your attention on your heart's recovery. Observe your breath as it gradually calms. Once you feel recovered and up to it, run another 10 steps and stop to recover. As long as you create a bit of an oxygen debt, your body will get the message and get to work at improving your ability to get more oxygen, more blood and more energy to your muscles. After a week, try to run 12 steps. It's the progression that counts!

Outdoor Running: Timed Exertion Periods

Warm-up	Set 1		Set 2		Set 3	
	Exertion	Recovery	Exertion	Recovery	Exertion	Recovery
1 min	2 min	2 min	90 sec	2 min	60 sec	2 min

Set 4		Set 5		Set 6	
Exertion	Recovery	Exertion	Recovery	Exertion	Recovery
45 sec	2 min	30 sec	2 min	20 sec	1 min

Like the distance program, start at a low to moderate intensity and increase the level of difficulty slightly after each recovery period. When you're running outdoors, you have an additional option beyond running faster for raising intensity - running uphill. Your local area and terrain will determine which will work best.

2. Treadmill: I'm not a fan of treadmills but if you can't get outside an indoors treadmill is a reasonable second choice. You can raise intensity via speed or incline at the touch of a button. You also have the option of holding on to the side rails if you feel winded.

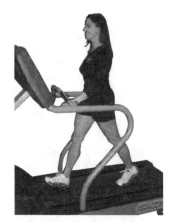

Begin walking at a comfortable pace for a few minutes until your muscles feel warm and loose. Increase the pace and lengthen your strides into a brisk walk, allowing your body to adapt. Start your first exertion period from this point. (Remember to wear proper running shoes with cushioned soles that absorb the impact of running.)

A sample treadmill PACE® program will look similar to the outdoor, timed interval workout above – with a few slight variations. Bear in mind that it's easier to run fast or sprint when you're outside. When on a treadmill, I find it necessary to start and finish with a longer exertion period.

Note: For treadmill programs, it is easy and works well to <u>increase the intensity</u> after each recovery period by slightly increasing your speed. After you have increased speed steadily over about 6 weeks, drop your speed back to your original starting speed but increase the slope and repeat the entire cycle with the higher slope.

Treadmill Workout

Warm-up	Set 1		Set 2		Set 3	
	Exertion	Recovery	Exertion	Recovery	Exertion	Recovery
1 min	3 min	2 min	2 min	2 min	1 min	2 min

Set 4		Set 5		Set 6	
Exertion	Recovery	Exertion	Recovery	Exertion	Recovery
1 min	2 min	2 min	2 min	2 min	2 min

3. Elliptical Machine: The elliptical trainer provides a high-energy, low-impact work out. This is a good option if you enjoy the feeling of running but don't like the pressure and impact on your knees. You also have the added benefit of cranking up the resistance to the point that stimulates significant muscle growth in the quads and glutes (thighs and buttocks). It can be very demanding with resistance. If you want to train your speed you can keep the resistance level low and really pour it on during the last few intervals.

Elliptical machines also allow you to concentrate your workout more on either the lower or the upper body. To work your arms, focus on pushing and pulling the handles; for more of a lower body workout, rest your hands on the handgrips, turn up the resistance and push harder with your legs.

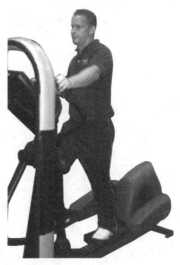

For this workout, I recommend starting out at no more than 2 minutes of exertion at a moderate level of difficulty. After each recovery period, increase the incline so that it takes more effort to run. You may want to hold on to the side rails for stability. Once you are used to this machine you can, for the last 2 exertion periods, run as fast as you can for 30 seconds each. You'll feel the burn in your thighs.

Note: To help you run faster, put the weight in the balls of your feet and lift your heels slightly. You can also raise your knees higher.

Elliptical Machine Workout

	Set 1		Set 2		Set 3	
Warm-up	Exertion	Recovery	Exertion	Recovery	Exertion	Recovery
2 min	2 min	2 min	90 sec	2 min	60 sec	2 min

Set 4		Set 5		Set 6	
Exertion	Recovery	Exertion	Recovery	Exertion	Recovery
40 sec	2 min	30 sec	2 min	20 sec	2 min

4. Stationary Bicycle – Recumbent Bicycle: When I'm in the gym, these two are my favorites. Both are great for working the larger muscles like the gluteus, quadriceps, and the muscles of the lower back.

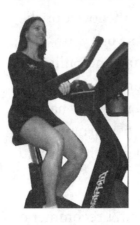 The stationary bike requires a little less effort, as your body is positioned over the pedals and your legs are pumping down. It also helps to improve your posture. Because both your hips and hands support your weight, your spine is in a horizontal position and gets a stretch in the lumbar region. The alternating hip motion created by your legs, works the muscles of the lower back, which affect your posture.

The recumbent bike is a good choice if you have edema (swelling) of the legs or problems with circulation. It also helps if you have lower back problems.

When exercising on a recumbent bike, you'll sit in a bucket seat and lean back against the backrest in a reclined position. The pedals on a recumbent bike are set horizontally in front of the seat, so your legs are straight out in front of you instead of below you. This puts less pressure on the joints, but makes resistance from the pedals a bit higher – giving you a more intense workout in a comfortable, natural position.

Stationary and Recumbent Bicycle Workout

This workout will challenge your endurance, so start at a low to moderate intensity. Increase the intensity as you progress. Feel the burn in your legs and take deep breaths making sure to exhale fully as the intervals shorten.

		Set 1		Set 2	
Warm-up		Exertion	Recovery	Exertion	Recovery
2 min		2 min	2 min	2 min	2 min
Set 3		Set 4		Set 5	
Exertion	Recovery	Exertion	Recovery	Exertion	Recovery
90 sec	2 min	60 sec	2 min	60 sec	2 min

After a few weeks, turn up the heat and try the following program. The intervals are a bit shorter, so you should focus on intensity and maximum effort.

		Set 1		Set 2	
Warm-up		Exertion	Recovery	Exertion	Recovery
2 min		1 min	2 min	1 min	2 min
Set 3		Set 4		Set 5	
Exertion	Recovery	Exertion	Recovery	Exertion	Recovery
30 sec	2 min	20 sec	2 min	20 sec	2 min

5. Outdoor Bicycle: Like outdoor running, you can vary your routines with both distance and time. To vary intensity, look for paths and terrain that go both up and down hill. You can use flat, straight-aways to work with timed intervals, increasing your intensity by going faster. Depending on your bike, you can also change gears to make it harder or easier to pedal.

The workout is similar to outdoor running, except the exertion distances are longer to account for the speed of a bicycle. Biking is ideal for overweight people because it is an exceptional fat burner and there is no impact to injure joints. If you will do this PACE® program and gradually increase the speed, you will get lean!

Outdoor Bicycle:
Brief Measured Distance Program

| Warm-up | Set 1 | | Set 2 | | Set 3 | |
	Exertion	Recovery	Exertion	Recovery	Exertion	Recovery
2 min	1 mile	3 min	1 mile	3 min	1/2 mile	3 min

| Set 4 | | Set 5 | | Set 6 | |
Exertion	Recovery	Exertion	Recovery	Exertion	Recovery
1/2 mile	3 min	1/4 mile	3 min	1/8 mile	3 min

Outdoor Bicycle:
Longer Timed Exertion Periods

| Warm-up | Set 1 | | Set 2 | | Set 3 | |
	Exertion	Recovery	Exertion	Recovery	Exertion	Recovery
2 min	4 min	3 min	4 min	3 min	3 min	3 min

| Set 4 | | Set 5 | | Set 6 | |
Exertion	Recovery	Exertion	Recovery	Exertion	Recovery
3 min	3 min	2 min	3 min	1 min	3 min

6. Swimming: This is a great way to practice PACE®. It works all the major muscle groups and gives your heart and lungs a good challenge. Swimming develops endurance, muscle strength, joint range of motion, lung power and improves posture and flexibility. Since the water negates the effect of gravity it's perfect if you're overweight, out of shape, pregnant or have mobility or back problems.

Swimming is one of the few "injury-free" exercises. Aside from the cardio-pulmonary challenge, you also get the benefit of resistance training. What's more, swimming does not put the strain on connective tissues that running, aerobics and some weight-training workouts do.

Because swimming does not involve the use of a particular instrument, like a bike or a fitness machine, you'll increase your challenge by either swimming faster or swimming a longer distance for each set and as you become conditioned over weeks of swimming with PACE®.

Swimming Workout

| | Set 1 | | Set 2 | | Set 3 | |
Warm-up	Exertion	Recovery	Exertion	Recovery	Exertion	Recovery
1 lap	6 laps	2 min	5 laps	2 min	4 laps	2 min

| | Set 4 | | Set 5 | | Set 6 | |
Exertion	Recovery	Exertion	Recovery	Exertion	Recovery
3 laps	2 min	2 laps	2 min	1 lap	2 min

The size of your pool will influence your workout. 6 laps in your own pool may be an appropriate challenge, whereas 6 laps in an Olympic size pool may be too much to start with.

Make adjustments as necessary. The most important thing here is creating the right challenge for you at your current capacity. During the last 3 exertion periods, you should feel your lungs expanding. Push yourself hard enough to initiate panting after each exertion period.

7. Jump Rope: This is more challenging than you may think. In fact, it's the best way to burn the most calories in the shortest amount of time. Skipping rope for just 10 minutes can burn between 100 and 150 calories (depending on the speed you skip and your body weight).

Once you learn how to jump rope with good coordination, you'll be able to skip for longer periods and tone your hamstrings, quads, glutes, and calves. Using a **weighted jump rope** is definitely not for the faint of heart. If you use even a 2 pound rope, your exertion periods will likely be counted in seconds.

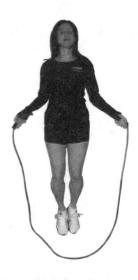

Jumping rope is also an ideal PACE® exercise and will push you to a higher fitness level. This in turn will help raise your metabolism, allowing your body to burn fat faster when performing less intense activities.

Skipping is convenient too. You can do it almost anywhere – in front of the TV, outdoors or in a hotel room – with little in the way of equipment. If you don't feel too silly doing it, it has a wonderful way of reminding you what it feels like to just play for the fun of it.

Exertion periods for jumping rope will be shorter than most. (Once you start, you'll see why.) If you find yourself getting tired too quickly, slow the speed of the rope. For example, instead of swinging the rope once for every jump, skip your feet 2 or 3 times – like jumping in place – for every swing of the rope. This will make it much easier to keep up. To increase the challenge, make short, fast jumps with a single swing of the rope for each jump during the later intervals.

You don't have to be anal about any of these routines. Instead of timing your sets, you can simply jump until you get tired, rest until you have recovered and repeat. Jumping rope is one activity that you may want to completely stop instead of just slowing down during your recovery periods. If you're not used to it, it's a bear.

Jump Rope Workout

Warm-up	Set 1		Set 2		Set 3	
	Exertion	Recovery	Exertion	Recovery	Exertion	Recovery
1 min	45 sec	1 min	60 sec	1 min	45 sec	1 min

	Set 4		Set 5		Set 6	
	Exertion	Recovery	Exertion	Recovery	Exertion	Recovery
	30 sec	1 min	30 sec	1 min	20 sec	1 min

8. Stair Stepper: Practicing PACE® on a stair stepper is not for the faint of heart either. But there are few other fitness machines that will pump-up the muscles of your lower body while providing you with an equally remarkable cardio-pulmonary workout in such a remarkably short time.

Stair steppers simulate climbing stairs. We all know how a few flights will make you out of breath when you didn't even know you were out of shape. The staircase has 8-inch stairs that rotate at pre-programmed rates. The rotation varies in speed to simulate fairly well walking – or running – up a flight of stairs.

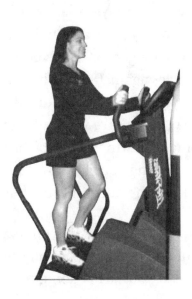

The stair stepper provides an excellent low-impact workout that particularly targets your glutes and calves. What's more, stair steppers are safe and put very little stress on your feet, knees and shins. It may not be the best if you have arthritis in your hips. If you feel, pain, popping or cracking in your hip joint, choose another instrument easy on the hips like swimming or a rowing machine. Stair steppers, when used with correct posture, are good however to rehabilitate an injured back.

For a high-intensity step workout, raise your legs at a 90-degree angle taking big steps, and only use the handrails for slight support. Leaning on the rails can hurt your posture and will lower the intensity of your workout.

Stand tall, with your knees positioned behind your toes. For the most difficult step workout, let go of the rails and pump your arms as you step.

Stair Stepper Workout

| Warm-up | Set 1 | | Set 2 | |
	Exertion	Recovery	Exertion	Recovery
2 min	2 min	3 min	90 sec	3 min

| Set 3 | | Set 4 | | Set 5 | |
Exertion	Recovery	Exertion	Recovery	Exertion	Recovery
60 sec	3 min	45 sec	3 min	20 sec	3 min

Take your first exertion period at a slow pace. Focus on your breath and pump your legs hard. Increase the intensity after every recovery period. You'll notice the recovery periods are a little longer for this exercise. You are using a lot of big muscles against pretty high resistance. This generates a big oxygen debt. Give yourself time at a leisurely pace for recovery. Make sure you make a full recovery (heart rate dropping to resting levels) before you start the next exertion period. During your last exertion period (20 seconds), let it rip and feel the burn in your thighs and buttocks.

9. Rowing Machine: This offers the benefit of a full-body workout with little impact on the joints. But don't be fooled; it's not just your arms doing the work.

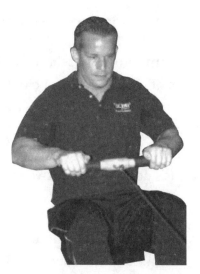

A good rowing machine simulates the experience of rowing a scull in open water. You glide back and forth on a seat as you draw the pulleys back in a traditional rowing movement. You can change the resistance and speed to fit your PACE® workout.

Proper rowing is an effective calorie burner and is great for "core" conditioning. It strengthens your arms, shoulders, back, abdomen and hips. Rowing has little to no impact on the joints, but you can pull the small muscles of your lower back if you're not careful. **Note:** It's important to keep your elbows close to the body.

Rhythm is very important here. It can give this exercise a relaxing almost hypnotic effect. This is one reason why I prefer slightly longer sets rowing. To increase the intensity, use the controls on your machine or increase your speed – especially during intervals 4 and 5.

Rowing Machine Workout

		Set 1		Set 2	
Warm-up		Exertion	Recovery	Exertion	Recovery
1 min		5 min	2 min	4 min	2 min
Set 3		Set 4		Set 5	
Exertion	Recovery	Exertion	Recovery	Exertion	Recovery
3 min	2 min	2 min	2 min	1 min	2 min

10. Trampoline: Trampolines are a fun – and effective – way to better condition. Yet they're not just toys. They're often used by professional skaters, dancers, divers, skiers and gymnasts to practice their turns, flips, and splits.

And the trampoline is great for PACE®. Children, seniors and adults new to exercising can benefit from the lower leg workout a trampoline delivers. The gentle activity of bouncing on a trampoline strengthens your voluntary and involuntary muscles, and helps your bones to become stronger. It's good preventative medicine for osteoporosis as well.

Achieving consistent height and balance on a trampoline takes coordination and lower leg strength. Compared to jogging or running on a treadmill, a trampoline reduces stress on your joints by 80 percent. And its easy and intuitive to start off with tiny bounces until you get conditioned and confident, providing an effective way to begin PACE® for older adults and those with physical limitations.

Mini trampolines – also called rebounders – are designed for exercising inside the home. Mini trampolines start at approximately 40-inches across – in square, rectangle, circular and octagonal styles. They're available in different tension styles: standard, super soft and therapeutic. For additional safety, many include a safety handrail that wraps around three sides.

For your PACE® routine, start slowly and focus on making steady, even jumps. To increase the intensity, jump higher during the exertion intervals and lower during recovery. For improving balance and coordination, focus on fluidity in your motion so there are no stops and starts. For greater stability as you jump, stretch your arms out to each side so that they're parallel to the ground – like wings on a plane.

Trampoline Workout

		Set 1		Set 2	
Warm-up		**Exertion**	**Recovery**	**Exertion**	**Recovery**
2 min		4 min	2 min	5 min	2 min
Set 3		**Set 4**		**Set 5**	
Exertion	**Recovery**	**Exertion**	**Recovery**	**Exertion**	**Recovery**
4 min	2 min	3 min	2 min	2 min	2 min

For the trampoline, longer exertion periods are more effective. Start slowly and accelerate as you move through each exercise set. During your recovery periods, bounce lightly in place and let your heart rate come down.

11. Calisthenics: It may not be an obvious choice, but you can do a very effective PACE® routine using calisthenics. You can focus on one single exercise (like Hindu squats) or combine several calisthenics into one PACE° workout.

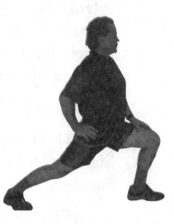

This puts all the benefits of PACE® and calisthenics into one, high-energy workout. It's definitely challenging, but nothing else will build muscle and burn fat so efficiently.

Calisthenics Workout

| Warm-up | Set 1 | | Set 2 | |
	Exertion	Recovery	Exertion	Recovery
3 min (Stretching)	3 min	2 min	2 min	2 min

| Set 3 | | Set 4 | | Set 5 | |
Exertion	Recovery	Exertion	Recovery	Exertion	Recovery
90 sec	2 min	1 min	2 min	30 sec	2 min

Begin with 3 minutes of stretching. Focus on loosening up the muscles in your legs and lower back. When you're ready, start your first exertion period. Let's say you're doing Hindu squats. Start at a slow to moderate pace – something you can sustain for 3 minutes. Stay focused on your breathing and make sure your fingertips brush the floor each time. (Refer back to chapter 6 for more details.)

When you're using calisthenics for PACE®, you'll adjust the **intensity** by speeding up or slowing down. So your first exertion period should be done at a slow to moderate speed. As you start each new exercise set, increase the intensity by doing it faster. By the time you reach your 5th exertion period, you should push yourself and by doing it quickly.

Note: Don't sacrifice precision for the sake of speed. It's important to practice calisthenics with the right form and posture.

Another option is to combine several calisthenics into one PACE® routine. Focus on calisthenics that build up the big muscles of your lower body like Hindu squats, lunges and jump squats. For each exercise set, choose a different calisthenics exercise.

3-Day Calisthenics Workout

While the big muscles of your lower body should be your top priority, you can also build a 3-day PACE® routine using an assortment of the calisthenics you learned in chapter 6.

Here's an example:

Day 1: <u>Lower Body</u>:
      Hindu Squats (2 sets)
      Lunges (2 sets)
      Jump Squats (2 sets)

Day 2: <u>Abs and Lower Back</u>:
      Crunches (2 sets)
      Leg Levers (2 sets)
      Scissors (2 sets)

Day 3: <u>Upper Body</u>:
      Push Ups (2 sets)
      Dips (2 sets)
      Instep Touches (2 sets)

12. Kettlebells: Kettlebells are balls of iron with handles. They were rediscovered in the US through the teachings of a Russian trainer named Pavel. He's a former Soviet Special Forces instructor and the trainer for the US Marines and US Secret Service.

Kettlebells are not for everyone but the results they produce are nothing short of electrifying. Once you try them, you'll quickly realize why the US Marines love them. (For more on kettlebells, check out: www.russiankettlebells.com)

Start with your feet shoulder width apart. Squat down and grasp the kettlebells. As you begin to stand up, swing the kettlebells out in front of you. As you crouch back into a squatting position, let the kettlebells come to rest on your forearms. Then push with your legs and stand straight up.

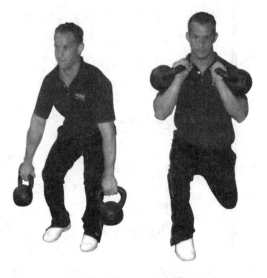

From this standing position, do a lunge by extending your right leg – then return to a standing position. Then do a lunge by extending your left leg – then return to a standing position. This series of movements is one repetition.

In your kettlebell workout below, each repetition will be referred to as a "rep."

When you apply this to your PACE® program, you'll do a series of these repetitions for each exertion interval.

Kettlebell Workout

	Set 1		Set 2	
Warm-up	Exertion	Recovery	Exertion	Recovery
3 min (Stretching)	5 reps	2 min	5 reps	2 min

Set 3		Set 4		Set 5	
Exertion	Recovery	Exertion	Recovery	Exertion	Recovery
4 reps	2 min	3 reps	2 min	2 reps	2 min

This workout is very challenging so go slow. Focus on your breath and your form. Pay attention to each movement. Don't worry about acceleration or increasing the intensity until you have enough experience and feel comfortable using the kettlebells.

Be Your Own Teacher:
Improvising with PACE®

These workouts are designed to give you a place to start. As you progress, you can increase the level of difficulty to match your needs and level of achievement.

You can do this by:

- Increasing the number of exercise sets in one workout.

- Shortening each exertion period and increasing the speed.

- Shortening each exertion period and increasing the resistance.

- After several weeks of the above, you can periodically reverse this strategy and drop your speed back to your beginning point, allowing you to lengthening each exertion period but this time with newly added resistance. (This will make the workout longer again, and give you more room to add other progressive elements later.)

Think of intensity as either speed, resistance or both, depending on the machine you're using. For example, if you're on a stationary bike, turn up the resistance to make it harder to pedal, or pedal faster or do both.

Remember change is key. Don't get stuck in a rut. If you're used to doing 5 exercise sets, add a sixth or seventh set to make it more challenging. **Don't be afraid to experiment but incremental change, a little bit at a time, is most effective.** The key to focus your effort on is not the routine but the change in your routine. Add some progression at least once a week. Change it up. When it feels routine, change it up again.

And, always strive to give your body a new challenge.

Doctor's Tip:

It is crucial that you have regular checkups, which could include mammograms, pap smears, checks for colon cancer, EKGs, etc. If you do not feel good, have your doctor check things out. If you are due for your annual mammogram, have it done. You could possibly be saving your own life.

CHAPTER 8

Reverse Disease with PACE®

P ACE® has such a direct and powerful benefit to your heart, lungs, blood vessels, muscles, joints, bones and hormones that you can use it to actually **reverse disease**. Asthma, COPD, heart disease and obesity are just a few of the afflictions I've reversed in my patients using PACE®.

In this chapter, I'll give you specific and detailed advice, along with customized PACE® programs to:

- Boost your lungpower

- Reverse heart disease

- Burn away excess fat

Pump-Up Your Lung Volume

It is almost impossible to overstate the link between your lungpower and your longevity. Simply stated, all other things being equal, the greater your lungpower, the longer you live. Did you ever wonder why so many elders die of flu and pneumonia? <u>By the time you reach 70 or 80, over half your lung capacity is completely gone</u>. And having no lung reserve power means you can't survive giving up any lung space to infection.

Mainstream Medicine Ignores the Facts: Lungpower is Essential to Good Health

I began to see the connection between lungpower and strength back in the mid-seventies. Later I became aware

---

of the pioneering work by Dr. Dean Ward in the 1980's connecting loss of lungpower to aging, the consequences then became very apparent.

This should have shocked the medical establishment... But his observation fell on deaf ears. To this day, mainstream medicine continues to ignore the vital importance of lungpower.

Smaller lungs mean a weak immune system and a loss of oxygen to your entire body. This sets the stage for sickness and disease. Look at this graph... By the time you're 50, you've lost 40 percent of your lung capacity!

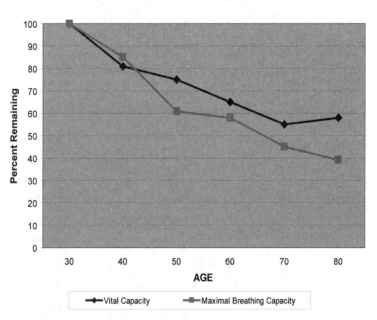

Age Related Loss of Lung Function

After twenty years of clinical research, it all points to the same thing: <u>Loss of lungpower spells bad news for your strength, your heart, your health, and your brain</u>!

- In 1988, the European Society of Cardiology reported that even a moderate decline of lung volume increases your risk of heart disease by 200 percent. This is true even for those who have no family history of heart disease.[1]

- In Denmark, the Copenhagen City Heart Study found that a loss of lung volume raises the risk of <u>first-time stroke</u> by over 30 percent boosts the risk of <u>fatal stroke</u> by 200 percent.[2]

- In the 1980s, Dr. Dean Ward compiled decades of studies showing that lung capacity is the <u>number one predictor of longevity</u>.[3]

Fine Tune Your PACE® Program and Boost Your Lungpower

As we discussed in earlier chapters, the key to expanding your lung volume with PACE® is creating an ***oxygen debt***. Let's review: An oxygen debt occurs when you ask your lungs for more oxygen than they can give you in that moment.

You'll notice this when you hit your recovery periods. After coming out of an intense exertion period, you'll start to pant. Every time you pant, you're triggering a response to increase your lung volume.

<u>When your body adapts to panting, your lungs get bigger</u>.

Let's say your using sprints for your PACE® workout. And each exertion period is a 100-yard sprint. If you're pushing yourself hard, by the time you cross that 100-yard point, you'll start to pant. The intensity of your sprint will determine how hard you pant after you finish.

For your first lungpower workout, try sprinting for 50 yards, then rest. Turn up the intensity and challenge yourself by running as fast as you can.

As you begin each recovery period, feel yourself pant. Are you merely breathing quickly or are you panting uncontrollably? <u>Strive to feel the panting as something involuntary – something that your body is doing to you</u>.

This is the point at which your lung volume will start to expand.

Recovery periods should last for at least 2 minutes in between exertion periods. Feel your heart rate recover and your breath slow down. When you feel rested, move to the next exertion period.

| Warm-up | Set 1 | | Set 2 | |
	Exertion	Recovery	Exertion	Recovery
3 min (Stretching)	50 yard sprint	2 to 3 min	50 yard sprint	2 to 3 min

| Set 3 | | Set 4 | | Set 5 | |
Exertion	Recovery	Exertion	Recovery	Exertion	Recovery
50 yard sprint	2 to 3 min	50 yard sprint	2 to 3 min	50 yard sprint	2 to 3 min

The idea is to workout at a rate that is very challenging for you at your current lung power but keep it brief during your exertion periods. By pushing your lungs to their limit, you'll start to pant. And that rapid-fire breathing will trigger chemical and hormonal changes that stimulate your lungs to grow and expand bigger, better and faster next time.

After doing the 50-yard runs at a moderate level 3 times a week for 2 weeks, try stepping it up to ¾ sprints. The challenge will be greater, but strive to run a little faster to maximize the demand on your lungs. After 2 more weeks start to flirt with all out sprints.

If this distance feels too short for you to create a good oxygen deficit that makes your lungs work at full capacity during the first 20 seconds of your recovery period, switch to 100-yard runs.

If you need you can rest for up to 3 to 6 minutes after each exertion. Again, feel your breath slowing back down. Feel the intensity of your panting. Allow your lungs to fill up and

Doctor's Tip:

Instead of taking an injury through rehabilitation after it is an injury, why not rehab before. You can actually take preventative measures before you indulge in a sport or activity by ensuring you stretch properly. This will help strengthen as well as stretch muscles, which in turn, helps reduce unnecessary injuries.

quickly empty. Feed your lungs the oxygen they need then remember to consciously blow all of your air out with each exhalation.

	Set 1		Set 2	
Warm-up	**Exertion**	**Recovery**	**Exertion**	**Recovery**
3 min (Stretching)	100 yard sprint	3 to 5 min	100 yard sprint	3 to 5 min

Set 3		Set 4		Set 5	
Exertion	**Recovery**	**Exertion**	**Recovery**	**Exertion**	**Recovery**
100 yard sprint	3 to 5 min	100 yard sprint	3 to 5 min	100 yard sprint	3 to 5 min

Not only will your lungpower increase, your breathing will become more and more relaxed. You'll start to notice that you take bigger, deeper breaths. You'll feel more power and greater endurance. Your mind will become sharper and your memory will improve.

What's more, you won't get sick as often – and I'm convinced that this may be the single most important tool for extending your "healthspan" that I can teach you. You may get years – even decades of added good health.

Patient Story: "RL" Boosts Energy, Lungpower – And Overcomes Depression...

When "RL" first came to see me, he complained of depression and lack of energy. What's more, he was carrying 39 percent body fat – almost off the charts. When I gave him a pulmonary function test, I discovered that he had limited lung capacity. Far less than I would hope to see for someone still in his thirties.

But within weeks of starting PACE®, he started turning things around. After just 3 months, he lost 18 pounds of fat and was breathing easier. Today, he's down to just 12 percent body fat. He's in better spirits than he's ever been, and his lung volume has improved to the point where he can actually sing.

(You may not realize this, but when the lungs are small and tight, good singing is almost impossible.)

Why Is Proper Breathing So Important?

Martial artists, yoga masters and high-level athletes from around the world have a secret weapon. It's what Bruce Lee called "Breath Power." The ability to control your breathing patterns to improve strength, stamina and sense of well being.

Besides delivering oxygen to your muscles during exertion, breathing is also the foundation for emotional intensity, physical equilibrium, and a sense of internal power.

Martial artists and high performance athletes of all kinds know that proper breathing techniques help them get in the zone, perform better and recover much more quickly. On top of that, improving your breathing literally helps improve your ability to develop higher and higher levels of functional fitness.

Dr. Alison McConnell, a researcher at Birmingham University, London, UK, says, "In addition to their role in bringing the air in and out of our lungs, the breathing muscles (principally the diaphragm, the muscles of the rib cage and the abdominal muscles) play a vital role in stabilizing and rotating the upper body."

So in essence, the quality of your breathing directly affects your core strength and lays the foundation for optimal athletic performance!

What Are The Benefits Of Proper Breathing?

Hundreds of studies have proven that proper breathing techniques before, during and after exercise delivers:

• Increased Stamina

- Increased Endurance

- Better Performance

- Quicker Recovery

- Enhanced Oxygen Absorption

- Increased Muscle Development

Proper breathing provides your body with oxygen for the correct and efficient functioning of every cell. Without sufficient oxygen, your muscles cannot perform at their peak, leaving you weak and listless part way through your workout.

Additionally, improper breathing inhibits your cells from metabolizing your food properly. That means all those nutrients and vitamins you need to build, tone and repair your muscles will be lost.

Proper breathing, on the other hand, allows your body to metabolize food efficiently and to rid itself of all the noxious gaseous by-products of metabolism, especially carbon dioxide.

Proper breathing soothes the nervous system; calms, steadies, and clears the mind; improves concentration; focuses attention; and increases the ability to deal with complex situations without suffering from stress. Plus, it tones and trains your diaphragm, rib and abdominal muscles to improve core strength and stability.

Basic Breathing Techniques You Can Use Today

Depending on whom you talk with there are hundreds of different breathing techniques to choose from. But for the sake of simplicity, we'll discuss four main breathing methods that have proven to help athletes improve stamina and strength.

Doctor's Tip:

When you stretch your body in preparation for exercise as well as after exercise, you need to stretch your mind as wellWhen your mind is relaxed, your body follows. To achieve a relaxed mind, listen to soothing music, relax your breathing, and use visualization techniques such as Yoga.

Focused Breathing — Most experts agree that for optimal health, your breathing should be full and rhythmic, using your diaphragm and ribs to fill and empty the lungs.

Your diaphragm is a large muscle that rests horizontally across the base of your rib cage. (Imagine an inflated parachute attached all around your lower rib cage.) The diaphragm is connected in the front, along the sides of your lower ribs, and along the back.

This type of deep abdominal breathing promotes a full exchange of air, keeping the oxygen/carbon dioxide ratio in your body balanced. Focused breathing utilizes this deep natural breathing pattern to develop rhythm and muscle focus while exercising.

Focused breathing should be deep and natural, with no impediments. The trick is to keep your mind focused upon your breathing and upon the muscles you are training.

For example, when doing squats, or deep knee bends you would inhale slowly as you descend then exhale as you rise to a standing position. You'll want to be sure to breathe in through your nose to strengthen your diaphragm and exhale through your mouth to alleviate pressure.

For pushups, simply inhale as you descend, exhale as you push your body up, using the same in through the nose out through the mouth technique described above.

Focused breathing is essential for proper development of your abdominals as well. Many people "forget" to breathe when doing sit-ups or abdominal crunches and lose much of the benefit of training. For maximum affect, inhale at your resting position and exhale as you contract your abdominal muscles.

To increase your benefits, sharpen your mental focus. For maximum muscle gain, focus your mind on the muscles you're training. See them contracting and relaxing as you rhythmically breath in and out. The connection between your mind and body while performing this breathing technique produces improved performance and overall muscle gain.

Using this focused breathing technique enhances your ability to perform each movement and will increase your fitness results over time.

Bellows Breath — The Bellows Breath is an adaptation of an ancient yoga breathing technique revered for its ability to increase energy and a sense of well being. Incorporate the Bellows breathing technique before or after your workout to improve cardiovascular function and to recover more quickly.

Begin by sitting in a comfortable position. Take a few deep breaths through your nose filling the lungs from bottom to the top -- like a glass of water. Expanding your abdomen and then filling the top of the lungs. Exhale through the nostrils doing the exact opposite. Expel the air from top to bottom, forcing the last of the air out with your abdomen pressing in.

After 2 to 3 warm up breaths, try blowing little puffs of air through your nostrils as you exhale. This should feel like a series of short, staccato exhalations, flexing your abdominal muscles inward with each short exhale. Be sure not to go to fast. After 15 to 20 repetitions, let your breathing return to normal.

The Bellows Breath technique will improve your stamina, overall concentration and sense of well being. It will "clear your head" and might even improve your cognitive abilities as well!

Lung Expansion — In this exercise, you will use deep diaphragmatic breathing to increase your lung capacity and to super oxygenate your muscles before and after a workout.

When you inhale, the diaphragm muscle pulls downward, such that the ribs flare out slightly, while the bottom of your lungs pull downward to bring in air. With deep diaphragmatic breathing, the space just below the breastbone, at the upper abdomen pushes in slightly to exhale more completely.

A Personal Story
By Usuff Omar - Sydney, Australia
As told to Dr. Sears' Staff

Dr. Sears' staff: Dr. Sears was happy to hear that PACE has helped you. But he is curious... What did jogging do to your heart?

Usuff: Jeff, I'd love to tell my story. I'm a 51 year old who has jogged with mixed results in the past.

In 2003 I started a new jogging program. After three months of consistent jogging I began to experience symptoms during and just after the jog that I now know (but didn't at the time) were of ischemia — the jogs became more and more strenuous, breathing harder to point of breathlessness, nauseous after jog, GI tract upset, felt faintheaded.

At the same time, off the jogging field, my heart would beat too fast for small stresses — emotional and physical. Walking up a slope, my heart would thump away (hey, with all my exercise, why is this happening? I'd ask.) My heart would race in response to minor emotional stresses too. It was an uncomfortable feeling.

The best description I can give is that my heart became 'elastic', easily stretched in terms of the HR escalating for the slightest reason. For example, once I took the garbage bin out and my HR watch I'd be wearing at the time would record something

---

incredible like 200 — huh? something is wrong with my polar watch I thought, as I didn't notice anything unusual. (I still don't know if it was my watch or me.)

Very thankfully, muscle soreness in my legs stopped me continuing to jog through my symptoms; shortly after that I read a connection between jogging and atrial fibrillation and immediately ceased my jogging program. My adverse symptoms gradually went away. That was in mid 2003.

However, my health was depressed in the remainder of 2003. Even felt depressed. But eventually recovered at the end of the year. An echo stress test in the beginning of 2004 proved normal, thankfully, and I was okayed by a cardiologist.

I tried to get an answer for what happened by asking an exercise physiologist on Allexperts.com, but didn't get an answer. For information, I put up my 2003 jogging notes onto a webpage for him, you might find it helpful. Its at:

http://www.geocities.com/usuff_omar/jogging2003.htm

In mid 2005 I felt some cognitive decline (probably from persistent poor sleep) and instinctively knew I had to return to exercise. This time I'd jog even slower. (In hindsight, insanity.)

I did, however, read in Dr. Kenneth Cooper's "Can Stress Heal" on page 84 that sprinting and periodic discomfort is good for you and felt it would be nice to incorporate it in future jogging — but was unsure how as I couldn't even handle slow jogging!

Luckily, before I could do damage to my body again from long slow jogs, I heard of the PACE program, and Dr. Sears' information on the dangers of long duration cardio. I knew I found the missing key. I began adopting a watered down version of PACE in April this year.

My jogs are now for 6 minutes, with three intervals, done three times a week. I'm increasing my duration/intensity at a glacial pace — I've learnt from my 2003 experience to gradually build up over months and years and carefully monitor for persistent adverse symptoms. (Another reason — my skeletal system takes longer catch up than my cardio system.)

I love PACE! Recently here in Sydney I had to catch a connecting suburban train which was arriving way at the other end of a very long platform. The train was pulling in and I had seconds to catch it. I accelerated and sprinted down that platform — a 51 year old man powering down like that, and without heart symptoms (no angina, little breathlessness) — I inspired myself, though missed the train.

I will be PACEing the rest of my life. The image of a 70 or 80 year old bursting into periodic sprints while slow jogging — an awesome vision.

Dr. Sears' staff: Also, can we use your story for future PACE articles?

Usuff: Sure, a way of giving back.

Dr. Sears' staff: By the way... Dr. Sears has a new PACE book coming out soon. It will have very detailed programs and insights. I think you'll love it...

Usuff: It will probably be my jogging Bible.

Please pass my deepest THANK YOUs to Dr. Sears. He has changed my life, probably saved it too.

Best regards,

Usuff Omar, Sydney, Australia

Inhale and exhale deeply pulling your shoulders back as you do. This will open up your lung cavity and allow your lungs to expand. Do 3 to 5 lung expansion breaths before and after each exercise to oxygenate your muscles and to shorten your recovery time.

Power Breathing — Use this technique to improve your actual strength while performing bodyweight calisthenics.

Unlike the previous forms of diaphragmatic breathing we've discussed, which require you to exhale completely, power breathing does not.

Power breathing is a method to increase the pressure in your abdomen to stimulate additional strength at the moment of exertion. If you've ever watched Olympic weight lifting or a martial arts competition, you've seen power breathing at work.

Here's how it works. Right before you perform a calisthenic exercise, inhale deeply through your nose. Be sure to breathe down into your abdomen and not just your chest. You'll know you're doing it right when you see your abdomen expand slightly as you inhale.

Next, hold your breath as you begin the exercise. Then as you begin to exert force, increase your abdominal pressure slightly. You'll probably feel the need to grunt, that's okay. Keep up the abdominal pressure through the full range of motion, then release.

There you have it. A quick primer on how to improve your breathing that will help you increase your natural stamina, strength and overall lungpower. Now let's look at how to improve our heart health.

SPECIAL NOTE:
Consult your doctor before performing this breathing technique if you have high blood pressure, heart problems, hernias or other health concerns.

Use Your PACE® Program to Reverse Heart Disease

To accomplish specific goals with your PACE® program, you simply create the right challenge so your body will make the right *adaptive response*. An adaptive response is simply the way your body reacts to a challenge. Simply knowing how to direct your body toward the right response will give you the results you want every time.

Creating an oxygen debt triggers the expansion of your lungs. For your heart, it's all about <u>heart rate and recovery</u>. You need to get your heart rate high enough to create the right challenge and then encourage a full and rapid recovery before you start your next exertion period.

Find Your Heart's Optimum Workout Level

We especially need a resilient heart today to handle the many stressors of our modern world. And even if you suffer from heart disease, you can reverse the symptoms and build a bulletproof heart that will take you to age 100 and beyond.

As we discussed earlier, most heart attacks are caused by sudden demands placed on the heart. That's why it's so important to condition your heart the RIGHT way. Building *reserve capacity* is critical. It's like having extra money in the bank that protects you from financial ruin. In this case, it protects you from dying of a heart attack.

As you now know, traditional training methods like durational cardio and excessive aerobic training can actually shrink your heart and reduce its capacity to adjust to changing demands.

But PACE® builds up that critical reserve capacity. Below, you'll find a PACE® workout designed to do just that. It's a relatively simple workout, but it has a twist…

Doctor's Tip:

Make it a daily challenge to find ways to move your body. Climb stairs if given a choice between that and escalators or elevators. Walk your dog; chase your kids; toss balls with friends, mow the lawn. Anything that moves your limbs is not only a fitness tool, it's a stress buster.

Instead of a recovery period that has a specific time limit, you're going to let your recovery period last for as long as you need to bring your heart rate down to your **resting pulse**.

Note: If you need to brush up on how to find your resting pulse, refer to chapter 4.

For your first heart-building workout, you're going to do exertion periods of one minute each. I recommend starting on either the treadmill or an elliptical machine. After each exertion period, I want you to rest until you hit your resting pulse.

		Set 1		Set 2	
Warm-up		**Exertion**	**Recovery**	**Exertion**	**Recovery**
3 min		1 min	Reach your resting pulse	1 min	Reach your resting pulse
Set 3		**Set 4**		**Set 5**	
Exertion	**Recovery**	**Exertion**	**Recovery**	**Exertion**	**Recovery**
1 min	Reach your resting pulse	1 min	Reach your resting pulse	1 min	Reach your resting pulse

During your first exertion period, start running and watch your heart rate. When you're in your exercise zone, hold that speed for one minute. After one minute, begin your recovery period. Walk at a slow, easy pace until you've hit your resting pulse. If you need to come to a complete stop, that's okay.

Watch the clock and make note of how quickly your heart rate goes from its exercise level down to its resting level. Write this down. As you improve, this number will get smaller. And the faster your recovery, the healthier your heart.

After 2 weeks, decrease the duration and start 50-second exertion periods. <u>But remember to increase the intensity level</u>.

This will serve you well the next time you find yourself in a stressful situation. When your heart is faced with sudden demands, that extra reserve capacity may mean the difference between life and death.

Melt Away those Extra Pounds: Use Your PACE® Program to Burn Fat

While lungpower and heart health are essential to life, fat burning and weight loss is the first thing my patients want to know about. Everyone wants to drop those extra pounds and hit their ideal weight. And with my PACE® program, I never disappoint them.

So far, you've discovered that creating an oxygen debt is the key to expanding your lung volume. Heart rate and recovery are the keys to heart health and reversing heart disease.

Intensity and **after burn** are the keys to fat burning. So forget about long, grueling cardio routines that last for an hour or more. To burn fat with PACE®, all you need is a minimum of 12 minutes – and never any more than 20!

In chapter 3, I told you about the clinical trial my Wellness Research Foundation recently completed. We put PACE® to the test by studying identical twins for 16 weeks. One twin practiced long-duration, traditional "cardio," while the other twin did PACE®.

At the beginning of the trial, both twins weighed the same and had almost identical body composition (same levels of fat and lean body mass). But after 16 weeks, the PACE® twin **lost twice as much fat**. Her body fat went from 25 percent down to 14 percent. She also gained 8 pounds of pure muscle, whereas the traditional cardio twin actually lost muscle.

Now it's YOUR Turn: Get in the Best Shape of Your Life NOW!

PACE® is the easiest and most reliable way to burn fat. Short, intense exertion periods will get the job done right. And it only takes minutes a day.

The trick is to trigger an "after burn." This happens when your body burns fat after you stop exercising. Here's the secret: It's all about what your body uses for fuel during exercise.

Remember our discussion from chapter 2… During the first minute or two, your body burns ATP (adenosine triphosphate) for energy. This is your body's most potent and available source of energy. It's used for quick bursts of movement, but it doesn't last long.

After a few minutes, your body shifts gears and starts to burn carbs in your muscle tissue. This lasts for 15 to 20 minutes. When you stop exercising during this process, your body will automatically burn fat to replace the carbs you just burned. **This "after burn" melts away the fat your body has put "in storage."**

<u>You'll continue to burn fat up to a full day after you finish each PACE® session</u>.

This is largely due to the boost your metabolism gets from your PACE® training. Because your body needs extra calories to repair muscles, replenish energy stores and restore your body to its "normal" state, you continue to burn calories – and fat – long after your workout is over.[4]

<u>After a few months of PACE®, your body stops storing fat because it simply doesn't need it</u>. This the opposite of what traditional exercise "experts" will tell you to do. Conventional wisdom tells you to burn fat during exercise. But this only makes matters worse.

Doctor's Tip:

Easier said than done, stress busters come in many forms. Some techniques recommended by experts are to think positive thoughts. Spend 30 minutes a day doing something you like. Soak in a hot tub, walk on the beach or in a park, read a good book, play with your dog, listen to soothing music, get a massage, a facial or a haircut.

This tells your body to make and store more fat so you'll have something to burn during your next workout. This is why so many people get frustrated when they don't see results after months of spending hours at the gym.

Turning up the intensity after each interval and keeping your workouts under 20 minutes will take your fat right off.

Your PACE® Program for Fat Burning

Warm-up	Set 1		Set 2	
	Exertion	Recovery	Exertion	Recovery
1 min	1 min	2 min	1 min	2 min

Set 3		Set 4		Set 5	
Exertion	Recovery	Exertion	Recovery	Exertion	Recovery
1 min	2 min	1 min	2 min	3 min	2 min

Before you start, choose your instrument. Running, either outdoors or on a treadmill works well for this exercise. But to really maximize fat loss, try a stationary bike or a recumbent bike. These will help work the big muscles in your legs. And by working those big – and often unused – muscle fibers, you'll enhance and speed up your weight loss.

During your first minute exertion period, start at a brisk pace and keep up that speed throughout. Follow the rhythm of your breath. That will help you maintain the intensity of each exertion period.

As you hit your recovery period, you should start panting. Allow yourself to breathe quickly and evenly, and focus on the feeling of your heart rate slowing down. After 2 minutes start your next exertion period.

As you begin your second exertion period, <u>turn up the level of difficulty</u>. On running machines, increase the incline so it takes more effort to run. On a stationary bike, increase the resistance to make it harder to pedal. You should immediately feel it in your thighs.

Continue with your PACE® routine, <u>turning up the level of difficulty after each exertion period</u>. By the time you hit your last exertion period, you should drop back the level but continue the last set for three minutes. That's all the duration you'll need to burn fat!

Learn to Generate Bigger "Heart Waves" and Beat the Diseases of Aging

Dr. Irving Dardik was the first Chairman of the US Olympic Committee's Sports Medicine Council, who made a Gold Medal winning discovery. This technique can actually reverse chronic diseases as diverse as Parkinson's, diabetes, multiple sclerosis and arthritis.

The story begins with Dr. Dardik's friend Jack Kelly. I told you this story earlier. (At the time, he was president of the US Olympic Committee. He went out for his usual morning run and, shortly after, dropped dead of sudden heart failure.)

Dr. Dardik knew that heart attacks often occur **after** running or jogging – not during the workout. He added that, *"People have been running for thousands of years, and they didn't die like that. It must be something in the way people run now that causes heart failure after exertion."*[5]

He also observed that long-distance runners were prone to infections and chronic diseases, especially heart disease. He compared their exercise practices to the habits of native people and animals.

He said that animals and natives in the wild run in short bursts. Then, they take time for recovery. And, they repeat this cycle of <u>exertion and recovery</u>. He concluded that long-distance runners die of heart attacks because they have not trained their hearts to recover. This is the same conclusion I reported in **The Doctor's Heart Cure**.[6]

Your Natural Heart Wave

These observations of cycles led Dr. Dardik to his fascinating concept of viewing heart exertion and recovery as a wave – the "Heart Wave." When you begin exercise, your heart rate begins to climb. When you stop, it begins to come back down. Think about that. If you plot these changing rates going up, then down, through time, it does indeed form a wave.

Inside that wave of exertion, you have smaller waves from each heartbeat – itself an alternating wave of exertion (systole) and recovery (diastole). Dardik was the first to see these as "waves within waves". The picture below will help you visualize the concept.

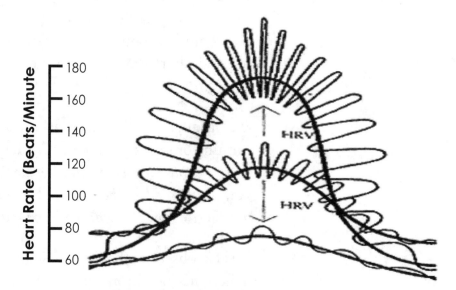

Heart Waves of health and disease: An expanding *Heart Wave* range corresponds to an increase in maximum heart rate and HRV (↑HRV) which promotes health while a decreasing *Heart Wave* range corresponds to a decrease in maximum heart rate and HRV (↓HRV) which promotes disease.

Generate Strong Heart Waves – and Reverse Disease

So why should you care? If you mimic the natural rhythms of your heart, and exercise in intervals of exertion and recovery, you gradually increase your heart rate variability, or HRV. Simply stated, the greater your HRV, the better your overall health. The more limited your HRV, the greater your risk of chronic disease.

In addition to increasing their heart rate variability, non-athletic women in Dr Dardik's study also gained:

- Greater Lung Volume

- Lower Blood Pressure

- Improved Immune Function

- Lower Stress and Anxiety

- Greater Sense of Energy and Well-being

All of these changes were in just 8 weeks. To quote Dardik, "Cyclic exercise really worked in reversing disease."[7]

Your 10-Minute Plan for Reconnecting to the Rhythms of Life

Of course, if you have a heart problem you should check with your personal physician before doing this or any other exercise. For this exercise, you can choose any activity that will provide exertion for your heart. A treadmill, elliptical machine, bicycle, jump rope, trampoline or alternating sprinting and walking will work well.

To maximize the amplitude of your heart wave, keep your exercise interval brief. Immediately upon finishing this brief sprint, put emphasis on your recovery. Instead of merely

Doctor's Tip:

Without proper nutrition and fluid intake, you can't have a great workout. Your body needs these fuels to build muscle and repair damaged tissue.

resting, participate in the process by calming your mind and imagining your heart rate slowing down.

To help with this, focus on each exhalation. As you breathe out, use your imagination to bring your heart rate down. In your mind's eye, see your heart relaxing – slowly and steadily returning to its resting rate. When your heart rate recovers, do another interval.

Here's a sample program you can do in about 10 minutes.

Warm-up	Set 1		Set 2		Set 3	
	Exertion	Recovery	Exertion	Recovery	Exertion	Recovery
2 min	1 min	2 to 4 min	40 sec	2 to 4 min	40 sec	2 to 4 min

Repeat this every couple of days but in the next session slightly increase the intensity. So if you're on a stationary bike, for example, increase the resistance a little each day so it's gradually harder to pedal. Now you are incorporating progressivity, a principle that Dr. Dardik neglected.

Any exercise you do will only continue to change your body through time if you incrementally increase something in the program.

By the time you've done this for 6 weeks you should be giving the 20-second interval all you've got then quickly changing your focus to recovering as fast as you can. This will focus your training on increasing your heart rate variability a most important cardiac capacity.

PACE® Yourself - For Life!

So now, you've discovered traditional cardio doesn't work, learned the fundamentals of PACE® and hopefully tried it for yourself. As you progress, you'll feel more comfortable monitoring your heart rate, creating an oxygen deficit and building functional strength with calisthenics.

But how do you make your dream of dramatic personal health transformation a reality? This where it comes to depend less on what you know – and more on *what you do*. I have done this for myself and in this appendix, I want to tell you how I made it happen.

Deep down, I know I'd be lazy if I allowed myself to be that way. My natural inclination is to procrastinate. But because I recognize this shortcoming, I've developed a system that makes health improving habits *automatic*.

If you will get started now and follow this specific plan of action… it will ensure that you don't put off your most important step – the actual doing.

Good Planning is the Key to Success

Every important accomplishment I have ever made started with planning. Every night, I take five minutes and plan my exercises and meals for the next day. I don't always stick to it, but without a plan, I tend to miss workouts and eat whatever is available. I don't bother with detail and I don't feel guilty if it changes. I think of it as a self-coaching tool.

Let's say tomorrow is Monday… I know I will be very busy with patients at the clinic and have several meetings afterwards. So I plan a brief PACE® workout before going to the office, and strength training at lunch. Otherwise, I know I'll never get it done.

For breakfast, I'll have eggs and some left-over salmon from tonight's dinner. For lunch, I'll order a seafood salad to-go from the restaurant near the gym. I take some steaks out of the freezer to thaw for dinner.

Guarantee Your Success: Keep a Record of Everything You Do

As a life-long "health nut," athlete, sports trainer, consultant, personal fitness trainer and integrative doctor, I've worked with thousands of people. I have found no better predictor of who will be successful at reaching there goals than whether or not they are willing to keep a log. <u>If you want progress, write down what you do.</u>

I have included excerpts from my own log below... I also use it for planning. I pencil it in and then write over it in pen when I actually do it.

Okay... enough talk. Let's get down to it.

Early to Bed, Early to Rise...

Ben Franklin was right. Getting up early is profoundly health enhancing. I incorporate this in my routine.

"6:00 AM: My alarm sounds. I put some motivation near the alarm the night before. Since I am in a leaning down cycle, I have my body composition log and my running equipment as the first thing I see. This makes it impossible to forget my goal and my motivation. I have a cup of coffee while I read my e-mail. It's now 6:45 AM and the sun is rising as I walk out the door."

I follow my PACE® program for cardio. As you already know, the principle is to build larger lung and heart capacity. To accomplish this, I provide my heart and lungs with short challenges just above my capacity to sustain.

When I stop to catch my breath, I know I've provided that little excess challenge. By doing this a little bit every day, I gradually build reserve capacity.

"Today I've decided to bicycle. I start with a 2-minute warm up at a gentle pace. I then accelerate to a moderate 5 out of 10 rating for 1 minute. I then drop back down to a 3 rating for 1 minute of recovery. I repeat this cycle 3 more times advancing to 6, 7, and 8 ratings for about a minute followed by a minute of recovery while I pedal at a 3 or 4 rating and breath deeply.

"Feels good today! For my last exertion period, I'm going to give it everything I have. I pedal as hard as I can for 30 seconds. I feel an intense burn in the front of my thighs as I move into my supra-aerobic zone. I know my body will get the message to improve my oxygen delivering capacity."

Warm Up	Set 1		Set 2		Set 3		Set 4		Set 5	
	Exert.	Rec.	Exert.	Rec.	Exert.	Rec.	Exert.	Rec.	Exert.	Rec.
2 min	1 min	1 min	1 min	1 min	45 sec	1 min	45 sec	1 min	30 sec	1 min

"I think about how important quads are to physical capacity as I am panting during recovery. "

Your quadriceps muscle is the largest in your body. It requires the most fuel. I pedal easily back to my house. Total time: 12 minutes.

Load Up on Protein for Breakfast

"Breakfast is a 3-egg omelet, salmon and water. I put 10 grams of glutamine in my water. It prevents muscle breakdown and boosts growth hormone. I take 1000-mg of Vitamin C and a combinational multi-vitamin, multi-mineral, multi-antioxidant supplement with my breakfast."

I have 2 basic rules to guide my eating. One, I don't eat food I don't like. I don't care who says it's good for me. Two, I try to eat only food that occurs naturally. Eating food that occurs naturally can be a challenge. Most modern food is man-made or adulterated in one way or another.

"After breakfast, I spend 20 minutes on calisthenics. First, I do one of my favorites, Hindu squats. To build strength in the legs and back – and boost your lung volume – this exercise can't be beat. Today, I'll just do 75 – although on some days, I'll push myself and do 500.

"I follow this with crunches, push-ups and instep touches. In just a few minutes, I've worked my entire body. As part of a regular routine, this is the best way to build muscle. It also develops the kind of functional strength that keeps you fit and mobile past 100.

"It's time to shower, and get to the office..."

Calisthenics Training Log		
Muscles Worked	**Exercise**	**Reps**
Legs, Gluteus	Hindu Squats	25 – 25 – 25
Abs, Lower Back	Crunches/Sit Ups	15 – 15 – 15
Upper Body	Push Ups	10 – 10
Full Body	Instep Touches	10 – 10

Reliable Energy for the Afternoon...

"I stop by a local restaurant and place an order for a seafood salad to-go. I ask them to add an extra portion of grilled salmon to the salad. Since I'm working the big muscles of the legs today, I want extra protein after my workout.

"I meet with my research assistant while I eat mixed seafood and spinach then it's time to see patients.

"After 2 hours of patients, I retreat to my office for a few minutes. I listen to music, drink a fruit smoothie and snack on some cheese. I finish with my patients, have a brief meeting with a perspective new employee for The Wellness Research Foundation and another with my office manager and it's off to baseball practice.

"I take the kids through some calisthenics. Exercising with 8 year olds has turned out to be great fun and I get to spend more time with my son. One hour to practice basic throwing, catching and hitting and it's home for dinner."

The Most Complete Nutrition Source

Despite the constant droning over the dangers of red meat, I eat it just about every day. In our natural environment, approximately 85% of our total calories came from red meat. Red meat is the highest quality nutrition – bar none.

In our modern world though, if you eat any animal you have to concern yourself with the environment of that animal. It makes all the difference in the world.

Keeping animals inactive and feeding them grains does the same thing to them that it does to us. It makes them obese with all the wrong kind of fat.

I much prefer **grass-fed** beef or wild game. It's full of heart-healthy nutrients with none of the hormones and antibiotics that can threaten your health. I have found wild game from a local hunting group. You can get grass-fed beef from my website: http://www.alsearsmd.com/content/index.php?id=114

"Today it's T-bones on the grill. I also grill up some onions and bell peppers. In Florida, we have tomatoes ripe now. I pick one yellow tomato and two red beefsteak tomatoes from my back yard. I wash and slice them and dinner is ready. I enjoy my steak and vegetables on the back patio with my family as the sun goes down.

"I take another 1000 mg of vitamin C and 400 IU mixed tocopherols with dinner. I also take 100 mg of Coenzyme Q10."

Mmm... Peaches and Cream

"I have a bowl of ice cream with a sliced peach, hand-whipped cream and walnuts. I don't worry about fat but I do try to eat low glycemic fruit. Peaches have a glycemic index lower than whole wheat bread. I also buy ice cream without added sugar. You can get it from most grocery stores."

	Meal Log	Supplements
Breakfast	Cup of Coffee, 3 egg omelet, salmon, water	Glutamine 10 gm Vit C 1000 mg Multivitamin
Lunch	Seafood salad with extra grilled dolphin and spinach	
Afternoon Snack	Fruit Smoothie, cheese	
Dinner	Grilled grass-fed steak, onions, bell peppers, tomatoes	Vit C 1000 mg Tocopherols 400 IU Co Q10 100 mg
Evening Snack	Bowl of ice cream with a sliced peach and walnuts	

Quiet Reflection...
Exercise for the Soul

Freud said we need three things to be happy: relationships, occupation and recreation. In other words, we need to love, work, and play. Under the stress of our modern lifestyle, we tend to focus nearly all of our energy for change on our careers. When that happens, we often neglect relationships and recreation.

I take a contemplative walk around my neighborhood. This is not real physical exercise and most people get plenty of walking during their daily routine but it does allow me to relax. Afterwards, I may watch some TV or read.

I think it is a mistake to treat your health and fitness goals as you do your occupation. I do not consider a health improving lifestyle to be work. It's part of my recreation. Plan it in the same spirit you would plan a mini-vacation. I also try to involve family and friends whenever possible.

"11:00 PM: Time to hit the sack. I think for a few minutes about what I'd like to accomplish tomorrow. What I would like to eat and how I feel about exercise. I jot it down in my log. I clear my mind and reflect for a few minutes. Now, I get to bed early."

Chart Your Daily Action Plan

- Make Your Plan for Eating and Exercise the Day Before.

- Focus Your Plan On Exercise You Enjoy and Eat Only the Natural Foods You Like.

- Start The Day Right With Brief Cardio Exercise Before Breakfast.

- Eat A High Protein Breakfast.

- Train for Strength either Before Lunch or Before Dinner.

- Make A Portion Of Your Physical Activity Recreation Every Day.

- Plan Dinner around High Quality Protein (Steak, Roast, Fish, Chicken).

- Involve Your Family And Your Friends.

- Reflect On Today's Progress and Plan for Tomorrow's.

I credit my good health to my daily habits. No one will ever convince me otherwise. But having said that, I don't beat myself up if I slip. I am not perfect and I suspect you aren't either. You won't succeed everyday and you shouldn't expect to.

Remember, excellent health is more of a journey than a destination. So be sure to enjoy the trip...

PACE® Q & A: Finding the Good Life the Easiest Way

Most people assume they have to overwork themselves to get results when they begin the PACE® program.

It's true that you will focus your attention on intensity levels while exercising... <u>but you don't have to work at uncomfortable levels to get results</u>.

Begin your PACE® program at a comfortable level for you. Continue to focus on increasing your intensity level, rather than the duration, as it becomes easier to do. By increasing the exercise level, you are adding heart reserve capacity.

A Steady PACE® Wins the Race

Success with my PACE® program is a gradual, week-by-week progression. As your body responds to the challenge, you increase the level of activity... without feeling an uncomfortable or painful perceived level of exertion.

It's important to remember that the reserve capacity of your heart, lungs, and muscles responds to as little as <u>ten minutes a day</u>.

At first, expect your heart rate to be at the lower end of the target range. As you challenge your heart a little more each time, as the weeks go by, you'll see that you're not only challenging its rate, but also its ability to rise higher faster.

Questions and Answers about PACE®

Readers often have specific questions that deserve serious answers. Many people will benefit from the following questions and answers about my PACE® program:

Q – Isn't PACE® the same thing as interval training?

A – No. Interval training has been around for about 70 years, but is simply running in short spurts with breaks in between. Most people who used intervals ran too long without adequate time in between, recovery was ignored and there were usually no progressive changes. For most it simply meant continuous exercise but at intervals of greater and lower intensity. This alone often made it better than continuous, steady-pace cardio, but my PACE® program is much more than the idea of intervals.

By adding elements of progressivity, acceleration, with gradually increased intensity and shortened duration, and the conscious feature of also training your capacity to recover from physical stressors after each exertion, PACE® enables you to avoid heart attacks, strokes, heart disease and reverse the effects of aging. These clinically tested facets of PACE® – which we don't find in interval training – produce dramatically different results when pursued over time.

Q – I am 74 years old and not particularly fit. Would PACE® work for me?

A – Yes, PACE® will work for you because you start with your current level of fitness. Over several weeks, increase your intensity. <u>The levels of intensity are what YOU define</u>.

If you're very out of shape, you can even do PACE® at different levels of *walking*. Walk at a brisk pace during your exertion period and walk slowly during your recovery.

Q – I always thought endurance training – like jogging and long-distance running – was the only way to keep your heart healthy. Why do you disagree?

A – What you really need is <u>faster and greater cardiac output</u>. By exercising for long periods, you actually induce the opposite response. You will do much more for your heart by exercising in brief spurts... ten minutes a day, if done effectively.

When you exercise continuously for more than about 15 to 20 minutes, your heart has to become more efficient. Greater efficiency comes from "downsizing." Remember, "smaller can go further." You actually give up maximal capacity with long endurance training.

Q – **My treadmill has various settings on it (1 to 10). Does that relate to the levels of intensity in PACE®?**

A – Yes, you can use your settings for your PACE® program. The intensity in PACE® is defined by your ability to do the exercise within you current comfortable level for a short time. But you can also increase the intensity level during your exertion period by simply running faster and/or harder – even though your machine may be set to the same number.

You can increase the incline on your treadmill to increase the intensity. So remember that intensity can be measured in several ways.

Q – **I'm in fairly good shape right now. Do you think I should do more than the 15 to 20 minutes you suggest – since I know that I can do it without difficulty?**

A – No, that defeats the purpose of the PACE® program. Instead of increasing the duration of your cardiovascular exercise, gradually increase some measure of intensity instead. Begin light and then pick up the pace or add resistance as your capacity increases. For your durational fitness use something more fun than cardio, like recreation or sport.

Q – **Can I do PACE® with other instruments, besides the ones you mention in your book?**

A – Actually, almost anything can be adapted for PACE®: Biking, treadmill, running, swimming... Even jumping rope or calisthenics. PACE® is very flexible. You could even do PACE® running up and down flights of stairs in an office building.

As long as you understand the concept of exertion and recovery along with progressivity, you can apply virtually any activity to PACE®.

Q – **In addition to increasing the capacity of my heart and lungs, are there any other benefits of short-duration exercise?**

A – Yes, there are several important benefits of short-duration exercising, such as burning fat, improving your cholesterol, boosting your testosterone and levels of growth hormone, working the larger muscle fibers, turbo-charging your metabolism and saving yourself time since you no longer have to spend hours in the gym.

Q – **Doesn't long endurance exercising burn twice as many calories – and lose twice as much fat – as short-term exercising?**

A – It seems that it should, but when researchers at Laval University in Quebec tested this, the results showed otherwise. By splitting participants into long duration and short duration groups, they found that the long endurance group burned twice as many calories as the short duration group. So they should have burned more fat, right? But they didn't. For every calorie burned, the short duration group lost 9 times more fat.

Remember, the key is "after burn." By limiting your

workout to 15 or 20 minutes, you'll continue to burn fat for at least 24 hours after you finish!

Q – **Isn't it true that long endurance training will protect me from heart disease?**

A – People don't have heart attacks from a lack of endurance. Heart attacks typically occur in one of two situations – either at rest or at periods of very high cardiac output.

We get a great source of data about heart health from the large Harvard Health Professionals Study. Researchers followed over 7,000 people. They found that the key to exercise is not length or endurance. It's intensity. The more energy a person exerted, the lower their risk of heart disease.[1]

High intensity exercise can also help you live longer. Another Harvard study compared vigorous and light exercise. Those who performed more vigorous exercise had a lower risk of death than those who performed less vigorous exercise.[2]

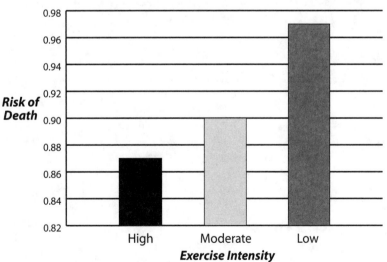

Exercise Intensity and Risk of Death

1 Lee I, et al. Relative intensity of physical activity and risk of coronary heart disease. Circulation. 2003 Mar 4;107(8):1110-6.
2 Lee I, et al. Exercise intensity and longevity in men. The Harvard Alumni Health Study. JAMA. 1995 Apr 19;273(15):1179-84.

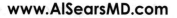

Charts and Forms

On the following pages you'll find charts and forms to use as you track your own progress with PACE®. You can either fill out the charts and forms here in the book, or photocopy them to keep handy for your exercise routine.

Heart Rate Journal

Date	Target Rate Range	Actual Rate

For more about the Heart Rate Journal, refer to Chapter 4.

Weeks	Warm Up	Set 1 Exertion	Set 1 Recovery	Set 2 Exertion	Set 2 Recovery	Set 3 Exertion	Set 3 Recovery
1 & 2							
3 & 4							
5 & 6							
7 & 8							
9 & 10							
11 & 12							
13 & 14							
15 & 16							
17 & 18							
19 & 20							

Weeks	Set 4 Exertion	Set 4 Recovery	Set 5 Exertion	Set 5 Recovery
1 & 2				
3 & 4				
5 & 6				
7 & 8				
9 & 10				
11 & 12				
13 & 14				
15 & 16				
17 & 18				
19 & 20				

For more about the Workout Chart, refer to Chapter 5.

Date					
Weight					
% of Body Fat					
Lbs. of Fat					
Lbs. of Lean Body Mass					
Max Heart Rate					

Date					
Weight					
% of Body Fat					
Lbs. of Fat					
Lbs. of Lean Body Mass					
Max Heart Rate					

Date					
Weight					
% of Body Fat					
Lbs. of Fat					
Lbs. of Lean Body Mass					
Max Heart Rate					

For more about the Body Fat Chart, refer to Chapter 5.

Week	Warm Up	Set 1		Set 2		Set 3	
		Exertion	Recovery	Exertion	Recovery	Exertion	Recovery
1							
2							
3							
4							

Week	Warm Up	Set 1		Set 2		Set 3	
		Exertion	Recovery	Exertion	Recovery	Exertion	Recovery
1							
2							
3							
4							

Week	Warm Up	Set 1		Set 2		Set 3	
		Exertion	Recovery	Exertion	Recovery	Exertion	Recovery
1							
2							
3							
4							

Week	Warm Up	Set 1		Set 2		Set 3	
		Exertion	Recovery	Exertion	Recovery	Exertion	Recovery
1							
2							
3							
4							

For more about the 12-Minute PACE® Program Chart, refer to Chapter 5.

Weeks	Warm Up	Set 1 Exert.	Set 1 Rec.	Set 2 Exert.	Set 2 Rec.	Set 3 Exert.	Set 3 Rec.	Set 4 Exert.	Set 4 Rec.
1 & 2									
3 & 4									
5 & 6									
7 & 8									

Weeks	Warm Up	Set 1 Exert.	Set 1 Rec.	Set 2 Exert.	Set 2 Rec.	Set 3 Exert.	Set 3 Rec.	Set 4 Exert.	Set 4 Rec.
1 & 2									
3 & 4									
5 & 6									
7 & 8									

Weeks	Warm Up	Set 1 Exert.	Set 1 Rec.	Set 2 Exert.	Set 2 Rec.	Set 3 Exert.	Set 3 Rec.	Set 4 Exert.	Set 4 Rec.
1 & 2									
3 & 4									
5 & 6									
7 & 8									

Weeks	Warm Up	Set 1 Exert.	Set 1 Rec.	Set 2 Exert.	Set 2 Rec.	Set 3 Exert.	Set 3 Rec.	Set 4 Exert.	Set 4 Rec.
1 & 2									
3 & 4									
5 & 6									
7 & 8									

For more about the PACE® 8-Week Intermediate Program, refer to Chapter 5.

Warm Up	Set 1		Set 2		Set 3		Set 4		Set 5	
	Exert.	Rec.	Exert.	Rec.	Exert.	Rec.	Exert.	Rec.	Exert.	Rec.

Warm Up	Set 1		Set 2		Set 3		Set 4		Set 5	
	Exert.	Rec.	Exert.	Rec.	Exert.	Rec.	Exert.	Rec.	Exert.	Rec.

Warm Up	Set 1		Set 2		Set 3		Set 4		Set 5	
	Exert.	Rec.	Exert.	Rec.	Exert.	Rec.	Exert.	Rec.	Exert.	Rec.

Warm Up	Set 1		Set 2		Set 3		Set 4		Set 5	
	Exert.	Rec.	Exert.	Rec.	Exert.	Rec.	Exert.	Rec.	Exert.	Rec.

Warm Up	Set 1		Set 2		Set 3		Set 4		Set 5	
	Exert.	Rec.	Exert.	Rec.	Exert.	Rec.	Exert.	Rec.	Exert.	Rec.

For more about the 5-Set, Short Duration, High-Intensity Workout, refer to Chapter 5.

Day 1	Set 1		Set 2		Set 3	
Warm-up	Exertion	Recovery	Exertion	Recovery	Exertion	Recovery

	Set 4		Set 5		Set 6	
	Exertion	Recovery	Exertion	Recovery	Exertion	Recovery

Day 2	Set 1		Set 2		Set 3	
Warm-up	Exertion	Recovery	Exertion	Recovery	Exertion	Recovery

	Set 4		Set 5		Set 6	
	Exertion	Recovery	Exertion	Recovery	Exertion	Recovery

Day 3	Set 1		Set 2		Set 3	
Warm-up	Exertion	Recovery	Exertion	Recovery	Exertion	Recovery

	Set 4		Set 5		Set 6	
	Exertion	Recovery	Exertion	Recovery	Exertion	Recovery

Continued on the next page...

For more about Extreme PACE®, refer to Chapter 5.

Day 4	Set 1		Set 2		Set 3	
Warm-up	Exertion	Recovery	Exertion	Recovery	Exertion	Recovery

	Set 4		Set 5		Set 6	
	Exertion	Recovery	Exertion	Recovery	Exertion	Recovery

Day 5	Set 1		Set 2		Set 3	
Warm-up	Exertion	Recovery	Exertion	Recovery	Exertion	Recovery

	Set 4		Set 5		Set 6	
	Exertion	Recovery	Exertion	Recovery	Exertion	Recovery

References

Chapter 1

1 From Wikipedia.org : http://en.wikipedia.org/wiki/Pheidippides

2 Liu M, Bergholm R, et al. A marathon run increases the susceptibility of LDL to oxidation in vitro and modifies plasma antioxidants. Am J Physiol Endocrinol Metab, 276: E1083-E1091, 1999; 0193-1849/99.

3 Hetland ML, Haarbo J, et al. Low bone mass and high bone turnover in male long distance runners. Journal of Clinical Endocrinology & Metabolism, Vol. 77, 770-775, 1993.

4 Press Release. Short bouts of exercise reduce fat in the bloodstream. American College of Sports Medicine. Aug 5, 2004.

5 Lee I, Sesso H, et al. Physical activity and coronary heart disease risk in men. Circulation. 2000; 102: 981-986.

6 Trappe S, Harber M, et al. Single muscle fiber adaptations with marathon training. J Appl Physiol, 101:721-727, 2006.

7 Van Helder WP. et al., Effect of Anaerobic and Aerobic Exercise of Equal Duration and Work Expenditure on Plasma Growth Hormone Levels, Eur J Appl Physiol 52 (1984) : 255-257.

8 Metabolism 1994; 43: 814-818

9 Medicine and Science in Sports and Exercise 2002; 34: 1468-1474.

10 Journal of Applied Physiology 1999: 87 (3) 982-992.

Chapter 2

1 Lee I., et al. Circulation 2003 Mar 4; 1087 (8): 2220-6.

2 Williams P. Relationships of heart disease risk factors to exercise quantity and intensity. Arch Intern Med. 1998;158:237-245.

3 Groscienski, Philip, MD, <u>Health Secrets of the Stone Age</u>. 2005, Oceanside, CA.

4 Tabata I, Nishimura K, et al. Effects of moderate-intensity endurance and high-intensity intermittent training on anaerobic capacity and VO2max. Med Sci Sports Exerc. 1996 Oct;28(10):1327-30.

5 Kolata G. Lactic Acid is Not Muscle's Foe, It's Fuel. The New York Times. May 16, 2006

Chapter 3

1 Nitti Joseph. The Interval Training Workout: Build Muscle and Burn Fat with Anaerobic Exercise. Hunter House Publishers. 2001

Chapter 4

None

Chapter 5

None

Chapter 6

1 Helliker K. Fears mount over dangers of pumping iron. The Wall Street Journal. Mar 13, 2003

2 "Understanding Calisthenics." www.humananatura.org. 2002.

3 Ross, Jill. Strength Training For Seniors. The American College of Sports Medicine. 2004.

4 "What Are the Specific Benefits of Exercise?" www.wholefitness.com

Chapter 7

None

Chapter 8

1 Cook DG, Shaper AG. Breathlessness, lung function and the risk of heart attack. European Society of Cardiology. Feb 29, 1988.

2 Truelsen T, Prescott E, et al. Lung function and risk of fatal and non-fatal stroke. The Copenhagen City Heart Study. International Journal of Epidemiology 2001; 30:145-151.

3 Dean W. Biological Aging Measurement –Clinical Applications. 1988. The Center for Bio-Gerontology. Los Angeles, CA.

4 Sedlock, Darlene, et al. Effect of exercise intensity and duration on postexercise energy expenditure. *Medicine & Science in Sports & Exercise*. 1989.

5 Lewin, R. Tuning Biorhythms through Cyclic Exercise. Holistic Primary Care. Spring 2006.

6 Sears, Al. The Doctor's Heart Cure. Dragon Door Publications, St. Paul, MN, 2004.

7 Lewin,R. Making Waves: Irving Dardik and his Superwave Principle. Rodale, 2005